the women's natural health series

Breast Health
the Natural Way

Deborah Gordon, M.D., Series Editor

DEBORAH MITCHELL
AND
DEBORAH GORDON, M.D.

A Lynn Sonberg Book

JOHN WILEY & SONS, INC.
New York • Chichester • Weinheim • Brisbane • Singapore • Toronto

Important Note

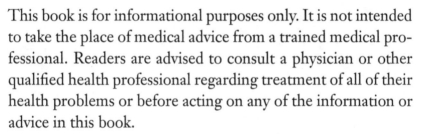

This book is for informational purposes only. It is not intended to take the place of medical advice from a trained medical professional. Readers are advised to consult a physician or other qualified health professional regarding treatment of all of their health problems or before acting on any of the information or advice in this book.

This book is intended to provide selected information about breast health. Research about breast health is ongoing and subject to conflicting interpretations. As a result, there is no guarantee that what we know about this subject won't change with time.

Contents

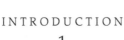

Introduction

By Deborah Gordon, M.D.

Rarely a day goes by that you don't hear a news report or read a newspaper or magazine article about breast cancer or about how some hormonal, environmental, genetic, or lifestyle factor affects women's breast health. There are studies about the cancer-causing effects of pesticides, how often you should get a mammogram, and the protective effects of vitamin D and sunlight. There are reports of breast implants gone bad and the increased risk of breast cancer from taking hormone replacement therapy. Additionally, you hear that a co-worker has just learned she has breast cancer, and that one of your best friends says she's changing to a cancer-fighting diet.

As a family physician who practices classical homeopathy, I see many women every week, some of whom are newly experiencing the changes caused by fluctuations in their hormone levels and others who are gracious, mature veterans of postmenopause. Every one of them, at one time or another, raises questions about her own breast health. Many of them are worried about how they can prevent breast cancer to the extent that some have a difficult time even approaching the subject. Others are concerned about breast pain and tenderness, the appearance and disappearance of breast lumps, and if they should breast-feed.

Even though heart disease is more prevalent and statistically a more deadly disease than breast cancer, the threat of the latter condition seems to loom larger and more insidiously over the heads of women everywhere. According to the National Cancer Institute, the risk of cancer grows dramatically as women age. Whereas a woman's chance of developing breast cancer is only 1 in 19,608 when she is 25 years old, it is 1 in 93 at 45 years of age, 1 in 33 at age 55, and 1 in 9 at age 85. (The 1 in 8 figure you hear so often is the risk at age 95.)

Whereas most people consider heart disease to be linked with an unhealthy lifestyle and thus a preventable condition, most women don't perceive breast cancer the same way. However, only 9 to 10% of breast cancer is linked with heredity and genes; the vast majority is associated with lifestyle and environmental factors. *This means you can do a lot, every day of your life, to help prevent this disease and to take control of your breast health overall.*

There is also much you can do to prevent recurrence and to live a full life if you should get breast cancer. Did you know that what you eat and drink have a tremendous impact on your breast health? Did you know that women with breast cancer are tapping into their mind/body connection to heal? Did you know that you can use Nature's remedies—herbs, homeopathy, nutritional supplements—to help you through radiation and chemotherapy treatments for breast cancer?

But this book isn't only about breast cancer. Many women come to me with questions about breast pain, tenderness, nipple discharge, breast-feeding issues, and other breast health concerns. How many women still believe that fibrocystic breast disease—that terrible misnomer—is really a disease and that it could lead to breast cancer?

The majority of the breast pain and tenderness, nipple discharge, lumps, and cysts that many women experience are related to cyclical fluctuations in hormone levels. Physicians who tell women they have a disease do a grave injustice to their patients. Those who take the time to explain hormone changes and related breast symptoms to their patients, and then suggest ways for coping with and managing those symptoms, allow women to take control of their breast health.

If you're a nursing mother, did you know there are herbs and homeopathic remedies, such as *Calendula* and *Pulsatilla*, that relieve breast problems associated with breast-feeding? Did you know there are herbs and nutritional supplements, including vitamin C and fenugreek, that can ease or eliminate breast pain? Have you ever considered taking the homeopathic remedy *Lycopodium* for sore, cracked nipples?

My role as a physician is twofold: (1) to thoroughly analyze my patients and select the correct homeopathic remedies that will improve their overall health; (2) to act as a consultant while providing women with the information and tools they need to be empowered about their health issues. This latter role is daunting, because each woman is unique, and there is a tremendous amount of information out there that can have an impact on women's health: from conventional to alternative medicine, from hard scientific data to anecdotal accounts, and from gold-standard treatments to late-breaking developments. I cannot hope to sit down and help each one of you sort through the wealth of information available. But I can steer you in the right direction and hand you the tools.

This book provides you with the information and the tools you need to take control of your breast health. Yes, you'll find information about routine breast examinations and mammography, but those things are only the tip of the iceberg when it comes to breast health.

I wish I would have had this book years ago to give to a patient like M.S., who consulted me after she had completed conventional treatment for breast cancer. Her primary concerns were depression, joint and muscle pain, fatigue, weight gain, and sleeping problems. Using a classical homeopathic approach, both her depression and joint and muscle pain improved significantly, and her fatigue was slightly better. As the pounds dropped off, M. S. began to experience menopausal symptoms, such as vaginal dryness and hot flashes, and her sleep disorder persisted.

At that point, we needed to do some significant research to decide which kind of hormone treatment, if any, might be appropriate for a woman who had been treated for breast cancer, while also taking into consideration her history and previous risk factors, current research on hormone treatment options and their risks, consultation with her cancer management team, and alternatives to hormone therapy. In short, it would have been very helpful to have had this book in hand. As it was, we decided to use small amounts of natural (oral) progesterone, which improved her sleep, eliminated her fatigue, and resolved her hot flashes.

Try as we may, we physicians cannot provide our patients with all the information and one-on-one attention they sometimes need. That's why I believe it is important for women to have access to timely, accurate information that can help them take control of their health as much as possible.

One of the most important things I do in my consulting role as a physician and as a woman is to help other women make friends with their body. Part of that friendship involves getting to understand their breasts: knowing how they function, what is normal and abnormal, and how to care for them in the most natural, safe, and effective ways available. To help you accomplish those tasks, this book offers a five-step program for breast health, along with comprehensive background and supporting information you can use to learn more about your breasts and to make informed decisions about your health. Here's a brief rundown of what you'll find in the following pages.

How This Book Can Help You

Your journey toward healthy breasts begins in Chapter 1 with an explanation of how the breasts develop and function, including the role that hormones, heredity, and lifestyle play in creating and maintaining healthy breasts. This is followed by a discussion of how women and North American society perceive the female breast and the emotional and psychological impact these perceptions have on women and how they care for their breasts.

Chapter 2 explores the changes a woman's breasts go through during pregnancy up to the time of breast-feeding. You will learn tips on how to maintain breast health and comfort during this important phase of your life. The chapter also offers guidelines on breast-feeding and how to provide optimal nourishment for your child; the use of medications or hormones during pregnancy and breast-feeding; and the positive and negative effects of pregnancy and breast-feeding on the breasts, including the risk of breast cancer, infections, and other complications.

Chapter 3 introduces the Five-Step Program for Breast Health and gives a brief explanation of each step and how the steps are covered in Chapters 4 through 8. This chapter also provides information on how to choose a health care provider.

Chapter 4 kicks off the program with Step 1: Eating for Healthy Breasts. A growing body of evidence shows that the food you eat has a tremendous impact on your risk of getting cancer and on maintaining breast health. In Chapter 4, you will learn about the healthiest options, focusing on the latest research from the American Institute for Cancer Research's Program for Cancer Prevention study. You'll learn the anticancer virtues of whole grains, fruits and vegetables, and soy products, and which foods are best if you are undergoing chemotherapy, radiation, or other cancer treatment. The health advantages of several other eating programs are introduced briefly, including the Gerson Diet and the Super Eight Food Groups by Dr. J. Robert Hatherill. To help you get started on a healthy eating plan, sample menus and recipes are provided.

Chapter 5 covers Step 2: Using Natural Supplements and Remedies for Healthy Breasts. It talks about the nutrients, herbs, and other supplements that can effectively reduce breast pain, help prevent breast cancer, and reduce the adverse effects of breast cancer treatment. It includes an overview of these beneficial natural substances and explains what they are for, how to take them, which forms to buy, and safety issues. If you have breast cancer, this chapter can help you choose natural herbs and supplements that can complement the conventional treatment you might be receiving.

Chapter 6 presents Step 3: Deciding If Hormones Are Right for You. The controversies and questions about the safety and effectiveness of birth-control pills, fertility drugs, and hormone replacement therapy are discussed. Every woman has taken, is taking, or is likely to take at least one of these types of hormones during her lifetime. Making the right choice can be confusing, which is why this step provides women with the latest information and guidelines in these three areas.

Chapter 7 addresses Step 4: Caring for Your Mind/Body. You know exercise benefits your heart, but did you know it's good for your breasts as well? In this chapter you will learn about the link between exercise and a decreased risk of breast cancer, the easiest movements to keep your breasts toned, and suggested exercises if you have undergone breast surgery. To help you reduce stress, which also decreases your risk of breast cancer, you can try the sample meditation and guided imagery sessions or learn about the benefits of yoga. You can also balance the mind/body connection by ridding your body of toxins that accumulate in the lymphatic system. This can be done

easily on your own through juice and herb fasts, herbal remedies, cleansing baths, saunas, as well as with lymphatic massage done by a professional therapist.

Chapter 8 explains Step 5: Breast Screening and Preventive
Maintenance. You will learn everything you need to know
about three important breast health measures: breast self-
examination, yearly examinations by your physician, and mammography, including some alternatives to mammography. Also
addressed is the debate about whether wearing a bra can cause
cancer, as well as tips on how to choose the most appropriate
and comfortable bra for you.

Chapter 9 explores the detrimental effects that certain
foods and food additives, alcohol, nicotine, caffeine, and environmental factors can have on breast health. Breast cancer has
been linked with various environmental pollutants, everyday
household products, and radiation and electromagnetic fields.

Your breasts are susceptible to various medical conditions,
most of which are not serious but can be painful or uncomfortable. The most serious condition is breast cancer, and
Chapter 10 presents an overview of what breast cancer is, its
risk factors, how it is diagnosed, natural approaches for how to
prevent it, conventional treatments, how to determine your
breast cancer risk, and the latest research on careers related to
breast cancer risk.

Chapter 11 looks at several less serious breast conditions,
including what is commonly called fibrocystic breast, as well as
mastalgia (severe breast pain), cysts, fibroadenomas, intraductal papilloma, fat necrosis, duct ectasia, sclerosing adenosis,
and various breast infections. You are referred to the appropriate natural remedies discussed in the Five-Step Program to
help you manage these benign breast conditions.

Sometimes taking charge of your breast health includes the
decision to undergo surgery. Chapter 12 discusses what to
expect when the breast is subjected to cosmetic surgery,

including augmentation, reduction, and lifts, and the options available to women after mastectomy or lumpectomy, which include breast reconstruction or prostheses. This chapter can help you make a decision about the procedure that is best for you.

I trust the information and suggestions you find within these pages will lead you firmly on the road to breast health and overall well-being. Of course, a book is only words. Only you can give those words power and meaning. Only you can take control of your health. Use these words as tools to make it happen for you.

CHAPTER ONE

Healthy Breasts: A Primer

Take a moment and think about your breasts. What's the first thing that comes to mind? If you are like most women, you have a definite opinion about them. And you're not happy. You think they are too small, too large, a bit uneven, or not firm enough. Many women define their sexuality by how their breasts look to them and how they think they look to their sexual partners. Surveys show that more than 40% of women, when asked how they felt about their breasts during puberty, reported they were embarrassed, shy, worried, or unhappy. Wouldn't it be wonderful if women learned at an early age to understand and appreciate this part of their anatomy?

Many women are afraid of their breasts: afraid of breast cancer, fearful of mammography, uncertain about how to examine themselves for lumps. They don't completely understand why their breasts go through so many changes every month and what those changes mean, except perhaps that they have something to do with hormones. They eye their breasts with trepidation whenever something "unusual" occurs, such as tenderness, pain, nipple discharge, or lumps, not knowing if they should be worried (in most cases, no, but you should be examined), and worrying nonetheless.

This chapter helps you replace worry with knowledge. With knowledge comes understanding, and with understanding comes the power to take control of your breast health. And that knowledge begins with the basics of breast development and function so that you can recognize what is normal, what is not normal, and what you can do about it.

Breast Basics: What You Need to Know

The female breast is the object of sexual desire, a source of nutrition, and a thing of beauty, but the anatomical definition is much more mundane: it is a modified sweat gland composed primarily of fat and glandular tissue. The size, shape, and health of your breasts are the product of your heredity, hormones, environment, and lifestyle. Heredity plays a large role in determining the appearance and health of your breasts. There's nothing you can do about your heredity: if your genes are coded for big breasts, you will naturally have big breasts. You can, however, have some effect on your hormone levels by controlling, to a large extent, your environment and lifestyle.

The Budding Breast

Female breast development begins in the womb at 6 weeks after conception. As the fetus develops, the female hormones estrogen and progesterone lay the groundwork for breast development. Estrogen stimulates the growth of ducts in the breasts, and both estrogen and progesterone promote development of the milk-producing glands, called lobular glands. At about the same time, the mother is producing hormones that assist in breast growth, including insulin, adrenal steroids, growth hormone, prolactin, thyroid-stimulating hormone, and luteinizing hormone.

The breast tissue, or mammary gland, is the first portion of the breast to develop. Along the area from the groin to just above the armpit, a parallel set of glands form on the fetus. This "milk ridge" disappears by week 9 of the pregnancy except for one pair of glands, which later develop into breasts. On rare occasions, one or two paired glands along the ridge remain, and an infant is born with an extra nipple. This is known as polymastia, and often appears as a mole.

Puberty

Aside from a slight nipple discharge called "witch's milk," which occurs in 80 to 90% of all infants during the first few days of birth, breast development lies dormant for the next 10 to 12 years. Then estrogen levels rise, which causes the hormone receptors in the breasts to stimulate the growth of the milk glands (see figure below). For some girls, this is accompanied by itchiness or slight pain under the nipple. This initial step into puberty typically begins before a girl's first menstrual period.

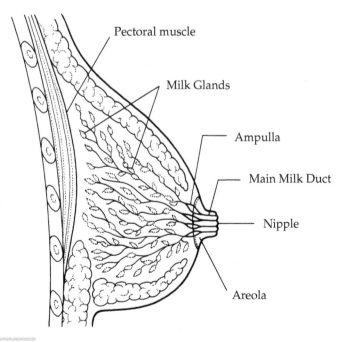

The Breast

Once menstruation begins (usually between years 11 and 15), a girl's breasts respond to the release of hormones from the brain, adrenal glands, and ovaries. Breast tenderness and swelling are the two most common symptoms during this time.

The Reproductive Years

Breast changes are associated with the menstrual cycle. When a young woman begins menstruation, all of the hormones involved in the process—follicle-stimulating hormone (FSH), estrogen, luteinizing hormone (LH), and progesterone—prepare the breasts for the possibility of nursing.

During the first half of the cycle, approximately 14 days before ovulation, FSH is released from the pituitary gland. FSH prompts the production of estrogen by the follicles, which are the eggs enveloped in a sac on the ovaries. As the blood's estrogen level rises, it causes the milk glands to swell, making the breasts firmer and larger. Once estrogen reaches a high level, FSH stops its work and LH takes over. Estrogen and LH initiate *ovulation*, which is when the follicle releases a mature egg. The second half of the menstrual cycle has begun.

As the egg travels down the fallopian tube on its way to a potential pregnancy, the ovary produces another hormone, *progesterone*. Progesterone prepares the breasts for breast-feeding and prompts the lining of the uterus to transform into an environment rich in blood vessels and glandular tissue for the approaching egg.

The most direct effect of hormones on the breasts is caused by the combination of estrogen and progesterone, which initiate an increase in ductal and lobular tissue, respectively. These changes result in the breast tenderness and swelling that affect many women during their menstrual cycle. They may also notice that their breasts feel lumpy during the second part of their cycle, which is normal. To alleviate any fear you have about these lumps, examine your breasts periodically throughout your menstrual cycle. If you notice your breasts are lumpy or lumpier during the second part of your cycle, you'll know the lumps are a normal part of your cycle.

If fertilization does not occur, estrogen and progesterone levels decline and menstruation begins. Without the high levels of these two hormones, breast swelling, tenderness, and lumpiness disappear. If, however, pregnancy is initiated, the breasts will undergo changes that prepare them for breast-feeding. Pregnancy and breast-feeding are covered in depth in Chapter 2.

Perimenopause and Menopause

For most women, their menstrual periods begin to change in regularity in their late 30s to early 40s as estrogen and progesterone levels decline. This period is commonly known as *perimenopause*. Internally, the supply of follicles is so low that they are unable to produce sufficient estrogen to maintain menstruation. As menstruation decreases (which often occurs gradually over months or even years), other body changes take place, including breast soreness and the formation of lumps or cysts in the breasts. Most of these lumps are benign and occur because the breast tissue shifts during this stage of life. (Chapter 11 discusses benign cysts and lumps.) Other symptoms of perimenopause include dry, flushed skin and backache.

Some women skip perimenopause and directly enter *menopause*, which is when menstrual flow stops completely. Unless you are on hormone replacement therapy (see Chapter 6), the dramatic decline in estrogen and progesterone causes the breast tissue to soften and thin. Fat then takes its place. Eventually follicle production of estrogen ceases completely and the role of the adrenal gland, which produces the hormone androgen (which is converted to estrogen), takes over whatever small amount of estrogen production occurs in the body. Around age 70, however, this alternate supply of estrogen also stops.

Variations in Breast Development

Female breasts can vary greatly in size and shape. The three most common variations are very small breasts, very large breasts, and asymmetrical breasts. All three types of development are the result of heredity, hormones, or both, and each can have a significant impact on your posture, how you feel about yourself, and how society views you. Other less common variations include amastia (absence of a nipple), inverted nipples, and extra breast tissue.

Very Small Breasts

The term "very small" is subjective. Although women with very small breasts can breast-feed and there are no physical or medical problems associated with having very small breasts, the psychological impact can be great. Some women who have very small breasts report feeling self-conscious, unattractive, and unappealing to the opposite sex. Women who want to change their appearance can wear a padded bra or may decide to have breast augmentation (see Chapter 12).

Very Large Breasts

On the other end of the spectrum are very large breasts. Some young women develop *virginal hypertrophy*, in which the mechanism that controls breast growth malfunctions and allows the breasts to keep growing. This results in a breast size that is out of proportion with the rest of the woman's body. Very large breasts can cause physical and emotional problems, including back pain, and the weight and stress of wearing a bra can result in painful indentations on the shoulders from the straps. Teenage girls with very large breasts are often the subjects of ridicule and ill-spirited gossip. Their size often makes it impossible for them to participate in sports or to dress like their peers.

Pregnancy can also lead to very large breasts, especially among women who are well developed before they become pregnant. Once the woman delivers, breast size may not return to the prepregnancy level. Women who gain a significant amount of weight may also experience uncomfortably large breasts. Many surgeons encourage weight loss rather than reduction surgery for these situations.

Asymmetrical Breasts

No two breasts in a pair are exactly alike. In some women, the cup size differs for each breast, which is perfectly normal. During adolescence this is often true because the breasts are still developing. Eventually, however, the growth rate generally evens out and the breasts are very similar in size and shape. In some cases, however, a woman's breasts are noticeably uneven. This can cause great emotional anguish for some women, in which case surgery—to either increase the size of the smaller breast or decrease the size of the larger one—may be an option. Specially made bras can make the breasts appear evenly matched under clothing.

Other Breast Variations

Inverted nipples, either on both breasts or just on one, are common. They are usually caused by scar tissue or other tissue from birth, although the inversion may not be apparent until the breasts begin to develop. Unlike breast size and shape, inverted nipples do make breast-feeding difficult (see Chapter 2).

A variation that often is not noticeable until a woman becomes pregnant is extra breast tissue, which is most commonly found under the armpit. Because breast tissue swells during pregnancy, a pregnant woman with extra breast tissue may notice swelling and hard lumps under her arm, yet it will not be apparent when she's not pregnant. This breast tissue can develop the same problems and conditions as normal breasts.

Women, Society, and the Female Breast

Throughout ancient times and up to the Victorian era, the female form appeared to be held in high esteem. Many art forms displayed the female breast either partially or completely uncovered, even among religious works. The Sistine Chapel, for example, depicts many bare female breasts. With the arrival of the Victorian age, female seminudity was quite acceptable in the art world, and in society women's clothing displayed much of the breasts. Voluptuous-looking breasts were much in fashion for several centuries, but in North America in the 1920s, a flat, boyish look became popular. This fad did not last long, however, and as the newly introduced brassiere became popular in the 1930s and 1940s, women's breasts were once again enhanced. It was during the second half of the twentieth century that the female breast became widely idolized.

Fueling the fascination with the female breast may have been the introduction of two icons: *Playboy* magazine (and similar men's magazines) and the Barbie doll. *Playboy* molded many men's attitudes about sexuality and the female body, especially the breasts. Part of the message sent to men was that young, firm, big breasts were the ideal. Barbie, with her sizable breasts, had the figure young girls were taught to covet. Thus, men knew what they wanted, and women knew it too. Advertising perpetuated the ideals. As media advanced technologically, it infiltrated every part of North Americans' lives, especially television, cable, and the Internet. Throughout it all, one thing became clear: sex sells, and young, big-breasted women really sell. The female breast became the symbol of female sexuality.

Despite the women's movement and cries for equal opportunity and against sexual harassment, most women still worry about their breast size. Evidence of this lies in the fact that approximately one million women per year get breast implants, and most of these operations are elective (unrelated to mastectomy) and for breast augmentation. So although most women may hate the fact that men have an image of the ideal female breast that women cannot fulfill, they try to fulfill it anyway.

Not every culture shares the North American attitude about the female breast. In much of the world, the female breast is respected for its beauty and its purpose, especially when it comes to breast-feeding. Among western European countries, topless beaches and public baths are common. Women in more primitive cultures, as in parts of Africa, rarely cover their breasts.

You've seen that your genes are responsible for the general appearance of your breasts. But there are other factors over which you do have some control when it comes to your breasts—factors that ultimately affect breast health including whether you get pregnant or breast-feed, your diet, how you handle stress, and how much exercise you get. If you are or plan to become pregnant, or if you plan to or are breast-feeding now, don't miss the next chapter. What you learn may ease any fears or questions you have about the changes that occur in your breasts during those special times, as well as help make you more comfortable and confident with those changes.

CHAPTER TWO

Pregnancy and Breast-Feeding

During pregnancy a woman glows—and grows—with the promise of new life. Her body also undergoes many changes. Many of these changes are linked to fluctuating hormone levels, which is certainly true of the effect pregnancy has on the breasts. As a woman's body prepares to give birth, her breasts also prepare to nourish her child. Mothers have long known that breast-feeding is beneficial for children, and research now shows that mothers get significant health benefits as well. This chapter explores the breast changes that occur when a woman is pregnant and breast-feeding and the effects those changes can have on her health and that of her child.

Pregnancy and the Female Breast

One of the first signs a woman has that she is pregnant is not necessarily a missed period; it's unusually tender breasts and/or nipples. This occurs as the levels of estrogen and progesterone begin to rise at the onset of pregnancy. Most pregnant women notice a significant increase in the size and firmness of their breasts within a month or two of conception, and some even say their breasts tingle. The nipples also enlarge and become erect, and the areolas darken.

In addition to outward physical changes, the body makes internal preparations for breast-feeding. Deep within the brain is the *hypothalamus*, home of the pituitary gland. This gland secretes two hormones responsible for milk production, prolactin and oxytocin. Levels of the former, which makes the milk, begin to rise at about the eighth week of pregnancy. Prolactin levels increase steadily but slowly until the seventh month of pregnancy, when they suddenly increase dramatically. The breasts swell further as the supply of milk builds in the *acini*, the glands that store the milk.

By the time a woman is ready to delivery her baby, most of the fatty tissue in her breasts has been replaced by glandular tissue. On average, each breast is about 1½ pounds heavier than it was before pregnancy. They will likely remain that size until she returns to her prepregnancy weight.

Once the baby is born, extra blood is sent to the alveoli. This causes the breasts to become very firm and full, and ready to deliver their milk. A detailed explanation of breast-feeding is given below.

To Breast-Feed or Not to Breast-Feed

Not every woman chooses or is able to breast-feed. If you decide not to breast-feed for personal reasons, or if there are medical reasons you cannot or should not breast-feed (see "Medical/Health Conditions That Can Affect Breast-Feeding," later in this chapter), you may experience some pain and discomfort during the first 24 to 48 hours after delivery. That's how long it takes for the body to recognize that milk is not needed and for the breasts to stop making it. Some women develop a headache, fever, and throbbing pain in their breasts and under their arms during these few days. These symptoms can be relieved by wearing a supportive bra, applying cold compresses to the breasts, and taking homeopathic remedies (see Chapter 5). Drugs designed to dry up milk production are not safe and should be avoided. A natural way to help dry up the milk supply is to drink 2 to 3 cups of sage tea per day.

Breast-Feeding and the Female Breast

Throughout a woman's pregnancy, high levels of estrogen and progesterone keep the flow of milk in check, even after the surge in prolactin production that occurs during the seventh month of pregnancy. As soon as the infant is born, levels of estrogen, progesterone, and prolactin decline, and the level of oxytocin increases, which prompts delivery of a premilk liquid called colostrum. This thick, yellow substance is rich in antibodies that help fight off infections and allergies, prevent intestinal problems, and build up the infant's immune system.

Preparing to Breast-Feed

Most new mothers feel awkward and nervous the first few times they breast-feed. That's because it involves positions, movements, and feelings that are new. Although it is not within the scope of this book to address all of the issues surrounding breast-feeding, this book does give you a solid foundation on matters concerning breast health. See Resources for sources of in-depth information on breast-feeding.

The Wonders of Breast-Feeding

When a baby begins to suckle, prolactin levels rise, prompting the production of milk. The nerves that surround the nipple and areola signal the hypothalamus, which then transmits a message to the pituitary gland to release oxytocin. The oxytocin stimulates the myoepithelial cells and the breast muscles to push the breast milk toward the ampulla, where the milk collects before it is released through the nipple (see figure on page 11).

The reflex that releases the milk from the breasts to the infant is called the let-down or the milk-ejection reflex. It operates automatically in the majority of women. It is often accompanied by the following signs:

- Tingling or mild pain in the breasts
- Appearance of milk even before the baby begins to nurse
- Uterine contractions
- Release of milk from both nipples at the same time
- A feeling of fullness or warmth in the breasts

The let-down reflex is intimately tied to a woman's emotional state. That's why some women find that they begin to leak milk when they hear their child cry or even when they think about their infant. The let-down reflex is an excellent example of the connection between mind and body.

Negative emotions or events can have a corresponding negative effect on let-down. Women who are experiencing pain, embarrassment, anger, fatigue, illness, or fear may find it hard to get their milk flowing initially. A trusted friend or a lactation expert from organizations such as La Leche League International and the International Childbirth Education Association can help in these matters (see Resources).

The American Academy of Pediatrics recommends that mothers breast-feed their infants for at least 6 months, preferably 1 year or longer. If you must breast-feed for a shorter time, do so while slowly weaning your child to formula. If you must return to work but also want to continue to breast-feed, use a breast pump and save your milk for your infant. Some mothers combine breast-feeding and formula feeding. Discuss your options with your doctor, or contact La Leche League International or the International Childbirth Education Association for more information.

SELF-CARE DURING BREAST-FEEDING

- Keep your nipples clean (do not use soap) and dry them after bathing and nursing to prevent cracking.

- Remember that whatever you eat is transferred to your child. The best foods are fruits and vegetables, whole grains, and other natural foods. Avoid processed foods; the additives and chemicals are passed along in your breast milk.

- Increase your food intake by 500 to 600 calories a day to provide nutrition for your infant.

- Drink plenty of liquids, such as fruit and vegetable juices, pure water, and herbal teas (no caffeine). Contrary to popular opinion, nursing mothers do not need to drink milk in order to produce milk. Avoid caffeine and alcohol.

- Avoid exposure to pesticides, herbicides, cigarette smoke, and other toxic chemicals, including chemicals used in cleaning products and those used to treat your garden. These can find their way into your breast milk.

- Take vitamins as recommended by your physician.

The Wonder of Breast Milk

The combination of colostrum and breast milk is Nature's most perfect food for infants to thrive and develop. Unlike cow's milk, which is uniquely suitable for calves, human breast milk, including colostrum, contains the specific nutrients in the proper balance designed for human infants. It takes 4 hours for infants to digest cow's milk but only 2 hours to digest human milk. Clearly the body must work harder to process a foreign substance.

During the first 4 weeks that a mother breast-feeds, the color and consistency of her milk changes as the percentage of colostrum declines and the amount of breast milk increases. At first, the mature milk is thin, like skim milk, but it gradually becomes thicker.

Breast milk is composed of a more nutritionally balanced combination of carbohydrates (mainly the sugar, lactose), protein, water, fats, vitamins, minerals, immunoglobulin (helps create immunity against disease), and cholesterol (great for infants, bad for adults). Recently scientists have discovered that breast milk also contains endorphins (natural painkillers), melatonin (a hormone associated with natural body rhythms), thyroid hormones, and growth hormones. The proper blend of nutrients derived from the mother's food intake is found in her breast milk because certain hormones, such as cortisol, insulin, and other nutritional hormones, specially process a mother's food and allow the right nutrients to become part of the breast milk.

Breast-fed babies typically do not gain as much weight as formula-fed infants, but this is not bad. In fact, breast-fed infants are generally much healthier than their formula-fed counterparts. Many Americans have the misconception that chubby babies are healthy, yet heavier babies are often getting more fat and less nutritionally dense foods than breast-fed infants.

The push to feed formula to infants has been driven by formula manufacturers who have a tremendous financial stake in perpetuating this practice. Although space does not permit an in-depth explanation here, many studies show both the health and financial benefits of breast-feeding over formula feeding (see Sources). Some of those benefits are listed below.

For Your Baby: Health Benefits of Breast-Feeding

One reason mothers choose to breast-feed is because it protects their infants against allergies, which is especially critical for premature infants. Research shows that preemies who are breast-fed have less than one-third of the allergies during their first 18 months of life. Here are some other health benefits for infants who are breast-fed:

- Higher antibody response to vaccinations. Infants who are fed formula may experience less protection from immunizations against disease.
- Colostrum carries antibodies to diseases the mother had before her pregnancy, such as measles, mumps, and chicken pox.
- Breast-fed infants are one-fifth to one-third less likely to die of sudden infant death syndrome (SIDS) than non-breast-fed infants.
- Reduced occurrence of diarrhea and vomiting among infants breast-fed for at least 13 weeks.
- Protection against infections from salmonellosis and giardiasis.
- Reduced rate of hospital admissions for gastrointestinal diseases.
- Less likely to be hospitalized when ill. Infants fed formula are 10 to 15 times more likely to require hospitalization when ill.
- Significantly reduced incidence (up to 83%) of necrotizing enterocolitis (a deadly disease of the gastrointestinal tract in infants).
- Protection against respiratory infections. Infants who are breast-fed are less than half as likely to require hospitalization for pneumonia or bronchiolitis.
- Significantly higher scores on cognitive development among breast-fed infants compared with those fed formula.

For You: Health Benefits of Breast-Feeding

Here are just a few of the many health benefits breast-feeding women can expect (for a list of 101 reasons to breast-feed, see the Web site www.promom.org/101):

- Possible reduced incidence of breast cancer (see section below).
- Reduced need for insulin among diabetic mothers who breast-feed.
- Lower blood pressure and levels of stress hormones, due to the hormone oxytocin, which is released during breast-feeding.
- Significantly reduced risk of endometrial and ovarian cancers.
- Protection against osteoporosis: a nursing mother's bone mineral density increases with each child she breast-feeds.

The physical and emotional bonding that takes place with the experience of breast-feeding is a benefit that is hard to measure. Other positive factors include not having to buy formula, knowing the milk is always at the right temperature, and eliminating the need to buy and wash bottles.

Pregnancy, Breast-Feeding, and the Risk of Breast Cancer

For many years, there seemed to be little debate about whether pregnancy and breast-feeding helped reduce a woman's risk of breast cancer. Indeed, many studies have pointed to a beneficial effect.

However, according to a study conducted by Patricia Coogan, M.D., and her associates at the Boston University School of Medicine in Brookline, Massachusetts, breast-feeding offers little or no protection against breast cancer. The researchers compared the breast-feeding histories of 446 women with breast cancer with the histories of 1471 cancer-free women. Both groups had a similar history of having breast-fed (83 and 85% respectively) and a similar risk of developing breast cancer. Earlier studies had suggested that breast-feeding reduces women's risk of breast cancer because estrogen levels are lower during lactation, and high levels have been linked with an increased risk of breast cancer. Dr. Coogan emphasizes, however, that breast-feeding offers "substantial benefits for infant health and therefore should be encouraged."

For now, the bottom line on breast-feeding is that even if it is proven not to protect against breast cancer, it certainly is not harmful. In fact, its many benefits, for both infants and mothers, far outweigh the few negative aspects, such as inconvenience or minor discomfort.

Possible Complications Associated with Breast-Feeding

Some women experience minor complications when they breast-feed. Below is an overview of the most common conditions and how you can remedy them.

Clogged Milk Duct

One or more milk ducts may become blocked during nursing. A clogged milk duct appears as a small, red, painful lump on the breast. You can eliminate the blockage by trying the following suggestions as soon as you notice the lump. It is critical that you continue to nurse. If you stop, infection may occur. Consult your physician if a clogged duct lasts more than 3 days:

- To relieve unnecessary pressure on your breasts, do not wear tight bras or other restrictive clothing, do not use nipple shields, and do not sleep on your stomach.
- To make sure all the milk from the affected breast has been eliminated after each feeding, hand express or pump the breast.
- Breast-feed more often and for longer periods of time. This allows your infant to better empty the breast of milk.
- If dried secretions form on your nipple, remove them gently with warm water.

- If clogged milk ducts are a recurring problem, consult a lactation specialist. Sometimes the way an infant nurses contributes to blocked ducts.

Cracked, Sore Nipples

Cracked nipples can be very sore and allow bacteria to penetrate the breast and possibly infect the milk ducts (see "Mastitis/Abscess," later in this chapter). One way to avoid sore, cracked nipples is to make sure the suckling infant places most or all of the areola, along with the nipple, in his or her mouth. Also prevent the infant from pulling on the nipple when he or she is removed from the breast.

Although some women use rubber nipple shields to prevent this problem, Dr. Eiger *(The Complete Book of Breastfeeding)* discourages their use. He notes that rubber and plastic nipple shields do not promote milk production and they rarely relieve soreness. Instead, treat sore, cracked nipples using the natural remedies explained in Chapter 5. Here are a few more tips:

- Do not use soap, witch hazel, alcohol, or tincture of benzoin on your nipples, as they will become dry and crack.
- Massage them with pure, medical-grade, anhydrous lanolin. It is safe to leave this type of lanolin on your nipples when your infant feeds.
- If one nipple is more sore than the other, start your baby on the less sore side so that he or she will be less hungry and less likely to suck hard on the second breast.
- Nurse more frequently but for shorter periods of time.
- Express a few drops of your milk and massage them into your nipples. Mother's milk has healing properties.
- Change feeding positions each time you nurse.

Engorgement

When a mother's mature breast milk first starts to flow, occasionally the breasts become so filled with milk that they become hard, swollen, and very tender, making them too painful to breast-feed. This situation, known as engorgement, can be remedied by expressing the milk by hand or by using a breast pump. Use one of the methods recommended below:

- To encourage the flow of milk, place hot compresses on the affected breast and massage the area with your fingers, pressing toward the nipple. These actions stimulate the release of oxytocin, which prompts milk flow.

- To hand-express the milk, support the breast with the hand corresponding to the breast. Place the tips of the thumb and first or second finger of the other hand on opposite sides of the outer edge of the areola. Squeeze your thumb and finger together using short, rhythmic motions. It may take several minutes for the milk to appear. Once the flow starts, work your fingers around the rest of the areola to help express milk from the other milk ducts.

- Keep your fingers on the outer edges of the areola; do not squeeze the nipple alone.

- To use a breast pump to express the milk, first massage the breast as noted above, then use the breast pump.

- To help relieve the pain, apply cold compresses between feedings. Homeopathic remedies are also effective (see Chapter 5). If these attempts fail, take one of the pain relievers identified as safe (see "Drugs Considered Safe for Nursing Mothers," later in this chapter).

Galactocele

Inflammation of the acini caused by clogged milk is known as galactocele, or a milk-retention cyst. This nontender lump does not become infected and rarely requires surgical removal. Once it is diagnosed by ultrasound or aspiration, a physician usually can resolve the cyst using needle aspiration.

Inverted Nipples

A woman with inverted nipples can still breast-feed. With the help of a simple exercise (explained below), the use of breast shields called Swedish milk cups, or both, an infant can breast-feed successfully.

The Hoffman exercise, which helps correct inverted nipples, can be started during pregnancy and continued throughout breast-feeding. Do the following twice a day:

- Place your thumb and forefinger of one hand or the index finger from each hand on opposite sides of the edge of the areola at the 3 and 9 o'clock positions.
- Press down and then stretch the skin from side to side.
- Hold for several seconds, then release.
- Rotate your fingers to the 12 and 6 o'clock positions and repeat.

Mastitis/Abscess

Mastitis is an infection of the breasts that causes them to become hot, swollen, and painful. It is caused by milk that becomes clogged in a breast duct, or it may be the result of an infection passed from the infant to the mother. If bacteria enter the duct through a cracked nipple, an infection can occur.

Mastitis should be treated immediately, because it can lead to a high fever, chills, headache, and an abscess. Treat mastitis or an abscess as follows:

- Apply hot compresses immediately before each nursing session.
- Massage your breasts.
- Express breast milk either manually or using a breast pump if nursing is not possible.
- Use calendula cream, vitamins, or homeopathic remedies (see Chapter 5).
- Avoid use of ice packs.

- Get as much rest as possible and drink plenty of fluids.
- As a last resort, use broad-spectrum antibiotics such as ampicillin, cephalexin, or erythromycin, which are not harmful to breast-feeding infants.

If an abscess does not disappear after treatment, it must be drained. Typically, physicians use an aspiration needle for small abscesses, or make a small incision for draining larger ones.

Mothers are encouraged to continue to breast-feed when they have mastitis, because it can actually improve the condition. In fact, many physicians recommend nursing every 2 hours around the clock. This helps eliminate the infection from the breast. Infants do not become infected with the bacteria associated with mastitis, because their stomach acid destroys the bacteria.

Surgery

Some breast surgeries can affect the ability to breast-feed. If you have had a breast lift, breast-feeding should be no problem. If, however, you have had a breast reduction or are considering it, you should know that about 50% of women who undergo this surgery are unable to breast-feed postoperatively. Thus, you may want to postpone this procedure until after you have nursed your children. Rarely, breast augmentation using silicone breast implants has caused infants to develop esophageal abnormalities, making it difficult for them to swallow.

Thrush

The yeast infection caused by the fungus *Candida albicans*, called thrush, is not serious, but it is contagious and can be painful, especially for your child. Your symptoms can include pink, crusty, itchy, or burning nipples; a vaginal yeast infection; or a burning pain inside your breasts during or after nursing. Infants may have white spots or a coating on their gums, tongue, or inside the cheeks. Some infants develop diaper rash whereas others have no symptoms at all. If you suspect thrush, call your doctor. The standard treatment for thrush is the prescription drug nystatin.

Use of Drugs during Pregnancy and Breast-Feeding

Women who plan to be or who are pregnant, and those who wish to breast-feed, should ask their health care provider about drugs, hormones, and herbs before taking them. Herbs, even though they are natural, are powerful and can affect your fetus and your breast milk just as medications can. Give them the same consideration you would drugs. For ease of discussion, drugs, herbs, and hormones are all referred to as "drugs" or "medications" in this section.

In many cases, the medications that can harm the fetus during pregnancy are much safer when taken during breast-feeding. That being said, you should be aware that there is much experts do not know about the effects of medications on a developing fetus and on nursing infants, largely because it isn't possible or ethical to directly test drugs on fetuses and infants. Thus, consider these recommendations before and during pregnancy and breast-feeding:

- Discuss any medication with your physician before you take it.
- Never take any drug unless you have a sound medical reason for doing so.

Here are some specific precautions concerning drug use during pregnancy and lactation. Consult your pharmacist or physician for additional details on these and other medications.

Drug Use before and during Pregnancy

Many people believe over-the-counter (OTC) medications are safe, and often that is true when they are taken as directed.

Before and during pregnancy, however, they can be especially dangerous to your fetus and to you.

Aspirin, for example, can increase the risk of bleeding for you and your fetus if you take full-strength aspirin during the last 3 months of your pregnancy. Women who take aspirin late in their pregnancy may experience a delay in the onset of labor, a reduction in the frequency and strength of their contractions, and an increase in the length of labor.

For OTC medications that are safe and unsafe for you and your baby, see the accompanying list. If you plan to become pregnant and are taking prescription drugs, consult your physician before you conceive.

The use of caffeine during pregnancy is controversial. Caffeine is addictive and can raise heart rate, increase feelings of nervousness and anxiety, and reduce your body's ability to absorb iron. It is a diuretic, which means your body loses vital nutrients (e.g., calcium, potassium, sodium, and magnesium) when you urinate. Caffeine also can cause temporary irregular heartbeat, tremors, and rapid respiration in the fetus. Some physicians strongly recommend that their patients avoid caffeine products; others say up to 3 cups per day is safe. Overall, however, caffeine has nothing positive to offer to your unborn child. Alternatives to caffeine-containing products are offered in Chapter 4.

SAFETY OF OTC DRUGS DURING PREGNANCY*

Unsafe

- Those that contain aspirin and caffeine, such as Anacin analgesic tablets, Excedrin Extra Strength, Vanquish caplets, and Cope.
- Nonsteroidal anti-inflammatory drugs (NSAIDs), which are believed to have side effects similar to those for aspirin. These drugs include ibuprofen (e.g., Advil,

Motrin, Nuprin) and naproxen (e.g., Anaprox, Naprosyn) and should be avoided during the last trimester.

- Cold medications that contain alcohol (e.g., NyQuil).
- Nasal sprays that contain oxymetazoline, such as Afrin, Coricidin Decongestant Nasal Mist, Neo-Synephrine 12 Hour Nasal Spray, and Vicks Sinex Long-Acting Decongestant.
- Antacids, such as Alka-Seltzer (types that contain aspirin) and Pepto-Bismol. Thorough testing has not been done on the newer antacids, such as Tagamet, Pepcid, and Zantac.
- Sleep aids, including Sominex, Sleep-Eze, and Excedrin P.M.

Generally Safe

- Acetaminophen, such as Tylenol. Although acetaminophen does enter the baby's bloodstream, it is safe in recommended doses. Continuous use of high doses, however, can result in birth defects.
- Antihistamines: Dramamine and Benadryl.
- Antacids: Maalox, Mylicon, Milk of Magnesia, Gelusil, Di-Gel, Tums, and Rolaids.
- Antidiarrheal: Kaopectate, Imodium A-D.
- Antifungal (for yeast infections): Gyne-Lotrimin, Mycelex G, Femstat, Monistat.
- Sleep aid: Unisom, but only infrequent use.

*For the latest information on substances that can harm a developing fetus, contact the Teratogen Registry at 1-800-532-3749, operated by the University of California, San Diego Medical Center.

Drug Use Before Breast-Feeding

If you plan to breast-feed, consider what effects any medication you take during labor and delivery may have on your infant. Anesthesia, including epidurals, pass through the placenta and enter the infant's bloodstream. Although your body can eliminate the drug within a few hours, a baby's immature system can hold on to the drug for weeks. If you receive a large amount of painkillers during delivery, they can make your infant sleepy and uninterested in nursing for a few days or longer. If you want to breast-feed, discuss the use of painkillers with your attending physician well before delivery.

Drug Use During Breast-Feeding

Whenever possible, first consider natural remedies rather than conventional medications when breast-feeding (see "Reduce or Eliminate Infant Exposure to Drugs in Breast Milk," later in this chapter). If you do choose drugs, Marvin S. Eiger, M.D., in *The Complete Book of Breastfeeding*, says, "You can safely take most commonly used drugs and continue nursing your baby." Dr. Eiger believes that, "All too often, physicians unnecessarily tell mothers not to breast-feed if they are taking any medicine, for fear that the substance will hurt the baby." Although many drugs do enter the mother's breast milk, not all of them have negative effects on breast-feeding infants. One reason is that the drug levels are generally less than 1 to 2% of the dosage taken by the mother.

This does not mean you have free rein to take high doses of a "safe" drug. The drugs in the list "Drugs Considered Safe for Nursing Mothers" can be taken in recommended doses and in limited amounts where indicated. Please consult your physician about any drug you want or need to take if you are breast-feeding.

Some drugs are known to be dangerous to infants and either must not be taken while you are breast-feeding, or you should stop nursing. These include chemotherapeutic agents (used to kill cancer cells), lithium (for bipolar disease), drugs that suppress the immune system, illegal drugs (e.g., marijuana, cocaine), and radioactive drugs used during diagnostic scans. Drugs whose effects are unknown include antianxiety agents (e.g., Valium), antipsychotics (e.g., Thorazine), antidepressives (e.g., Prozac), and some antibiotics (e.g., ciprofloxacin and chloramphenicol).

Nicotine interferes with milk production and can make your infant fretful. The debate over the effects of alcohol on breast-feeding infants is ongoing. The latest consensus is that binge drinking and daily consumption of one to two drinks are both harmful to nursing infants. La Leche League International reports that it takes up to 13 hours for a 120-pound woman to eliminate the alcohol from one drink from her body. Dr. Marianne Neifert (*Dr. Mom's Guide to Breastfeeding*) recommends not breast-feeding for at least 2 hours per drink consumed and to limit alcohol consumption to two drinks per week.

For the latest information on which medications are safe to take while breast-feeding, see the organizations and help lines listed in the Resources section at the back of this book.

DRUGS CONSIDERED SAFE FOR NURSING MOTHERS

Acetaminophen (Tylenol and others)

Acyclovir (for herpes)

Antacids (Maalox, Tums, and others)

Antibiotics (not all; check with physician)

Antiepileptic drugs

Antihypertensives (some beta-blockers are not safe; consult your physician)

Aspirin (one to two tablets daily for a few days; ibuprofen is preferred)

Caffeine (in moderation: Marianne Neifert, M.D., author of *Dr. Mom's Guide to Breastfeeding*, recommends no more than two cups of a caffeine beverage daily)

Cimetidine (Tagamet)

Codeine

Cold and flu remedies (over-the-counter)

Decongestants

Fluconazole (Diflucan)

Ibuprofen (Advil and others; use for only a few days)

Loperamide (Imodium)

Oral contraceptives (estrogens can reduce milk production; progestin-only have no effect)

Phenobarbital (very low doses only)

Prednisone

Tolbutamide (for diabetes)

Vaccines

*When taken as directed and with the knowledge of your physician.

Reduce or Eliminate Infant Exposure to Drugs in Breast Milk

Before you reach for that laxative, cold remedy, or headache pill, consider an alternative, nondrug method to relieve your symptoms. If you are experiencing constipation, for example, add more fiber to your diet and drink at least eight glasses of water a day. Rather than a decongestant, try steam treatments with a humidifier. Many headaches can be tamed with deep breathing, ice packs, and meditation. Muscle pain often responds to cold or hot compresses or massage.

The form of medication you take affects how much of it enters your breast milk. Capsules, tablets, and other ingested forms send higher levels of drugs to your breast milk than do lozenges, nose drops, and gargles.

Although herbal or nutritional supplements are often much safer than conventional drug treatments, do not assume they will have no effect on your infant. Always check with your physician or pharmacist before you take any natural remedies.

When you take a medication affects how much drug reaches your infant. Breast-feed immediately before you are scheduled to take a medication, because its level in your body will be at its lowest point. You can also take a dose before your infant's longest sleep period, which gives the drug time to clear your body. Avoid sustained-release or long-acting medications (e.g., those you take every 12 hours) because they stay in your system longer.

Medical/Health Conditions That Can Affect Breast-Feeding

Sometimes breast-feeding is not feasible or recommended because of a woman's medical condition or because of drugs or therapy she is taking. If you are undergoing chemotherapy, or if you are taking radioactive compounds (for example, gallium-67, iodine, or technetium-99m), lithium, ergotamine, or any recreational drugs, these harmful substances can be transmitted to your infant through your breast milk.

If you must receive radioactive agents, you can take a brief "vacation" from breast-feeding until the substance clears from your body. Depending on the agent used, this can take from 1 day to several weeks, although most drugs clear within a few days. To maintain milk production, express your milk and freeze it. This milk is safe to use because radioactivity disappears from the milk within hours or days, depending on the treatment and dosage used.

If you have human immunodeficiency virus (HIV) or acquired immunodeficiency syndrome (AIDS), breast-feeding is contraindicated. You can probably breast-feed if you have chronic hepatitis C, but consult your physician first. If you have hepatitis B, you can breast-feed if your infant received the hepatitis B vaccine within the first few days after birth. Women with untreated tuberculosis should not breast-feed until they have begun treatment.

Breast-Feeding and Minor Illnesses

If you have a cold, the flu, or a bacterial infection, continue to breast-feed, because once you have symptoms of an illness, your baby has already been exposed. By allowing your infant to breast-feed, he or she will get the benefit of the antibodies your body produces to fight off the illness. If you stop breast-feeding, you increase your infant's chances of getting sick.

Weaning and Breast Changes

When you stop breast-feeding, your hormone levels will return to pre-breast-feeding levels, and your body will undergo several changes. If you wean your child slowly, your milk production should decline steadily as well, although it may take several months before it disappears completely. During that time, stimulation of the nipples, such as during sexual activity, can cause some milk to leak. If you experience breast pain or discomfort during weaning because you are holding too much milk, hand express small amounts or allow your child to feed for a minute or two. Avoid releasing too much milk, however, because it will encourage more milk production.

It may take several months for your breasts to return to their prepregnancy size. Some women's breasts become larger and firmer after breast-feeding; others become smaller. Much depends on how much weight you've gained or lost.

Pregnancy and breast-feeding are two of the most natural stages of a woman's life, and they also involve many changes in the breasts. This chapter has introduced you to many of those changes so that you can better understand them and deal with them in ways that promote breast health. Now let's launch into the core of the book: the Five-Step Program for Breast Health.

CHAPTER THREE

Your Five-Step Program for Breast Health

Two of the most exciting things about health care today are the number of options for taking control of your own health needs and the vast amount of information available about those options. Often, however, the sheer volume of data, along with our busy lifestyles, makes it difficult to collect what we need and to assemble it into a usable form.

That's why the Five-Step Program for Breast Health was developed: for you and other busy women who want to take care of their breasts and who deserve to have the best informational tools within easy reach. The Five-Step Program includes actions all women can and should take to help ensure breast health. It is an easy, workable plan that offers you optimal protection with minimal effort. It puts control of your breast health where it should be: in your hands. True, this program is not a guarantee that you will not develop cysts, breast infections, or even breast cancer. But it does provide you with the guidelines and the knowledge you need to take care of your breasts and to have an appreciation for your body and your breasts.

You may already be following some of the guidelines, in which case implementing the entire program will be even easier. Regardless of where you are now, every step you take brings you closer to better health. These steps are recommendations only and should be used in conjunction with the advice of your physician or other health care provider. That being said, first you need to choose a physician or health care provider who will help you with your health and wellness goals.

How to Choose a Doctor or Other Health Care Provider

Every woman needs to have a physician or other health care practitioner whom she can turn to with confidence, not only if things go wrong, but also when she needs a few words of advice or guidance concerning her health. Selecting such a practitioner is a vital part of your program.

The following suggestions can help you choose a physician with whom you feel comfortable and with whom you can establish a good relationship. Keep in mind that it is a relationship, which means each of you is responsible for sharing information, asking questions, being open to new ideas, and being willing to learn. You may need the services of more than one health care provider—say, a medical doctor and one or more alternative practitioners who are knowledgeable about natural therapies. It is then your responsibility to let each health team member know what is taking place with the others. Your medical doctor, for example, needs to know if you are on an herbal program with your naturopath, because herbs may impact any medications prescribed by your physician. Conversely, conventional drugs can influence the effects of herbal remedies.

More and more physicians are receiving training in alternative therapies. It is not uncommon to find a medical doctor who also offers homeopathic care, nutritional therapy, or acupuncture. Even so, you may still want to consult an alternative health practitioner for other therapies.

Guidelines for Choosing a Physician/Health Care Practitioner

When considering candidates to be your health care provider, consider the following guidelines and questions:

- Get referrals from family, friends, and other trusted individuals. Because everyone has different priorities and tastes, ask these people why they like their practitioners. Their reasons may not meet your criteria.

- Do you want a male or female doctor? Many women prefer female doctors; others don't have a preference as long as the individual fits their needs.

- How do these health care providers feel about alternative or complementary therapies? Do they incorporate any natural therapies in their practice, or are they comfortable with patients who seek help from alternative practitioners?

- What are their feelings about the roles of nutrition and stress in overall health?

- What is their education and training background? Are they board certified? Check these facts by contacting the American Medical Association (www.ama-assn.org) and the American Board of Medical Specialties (800-776-2378; www.certifieddoctor.com).

- Are these health care providers willing to make referrals to specialists or other practitioners?

- Are they associated with a hospital, medical center, or clinic? If you ever require the services of one of these places, you need to be comfortable with the choice.

- Do they have diagnostic facilities, such as x-rays and a lab, on site? Having these services readily available is convenient for you when tests are needed.

- How do their offices handle insurance claims?
- Are their offices convenient for you?

Once you have narrowed down your choice, interview the health care provider to determine if he or she is the right one for you. Trust your gut instincts as you listen to the answers this person gives you:

- Does she or he answer your questions honestly and openly?
- Does she or he seem genuinely interested in your concerns?
- Does she or he take her time or does she seem impatient or rushed?
- How does she or he interact with her staff?
- Does she or he have another physician on call when she or he is unavailable?

If her or his answers satisfy you, congratulations! You have the makings of a relationship with your health care provider.

The Five-Step Program for Breast Health: An Overview

Step 1: Eating for Healthy Breasts

Perhaps you are already eating more fruits and vegetables, avoiding processed foods, including whole grains and beans in your diet, and enjoying soy products. Or you may be thinking about it but haven't yet made any changes. Now's the time to do it, and this step explains the why and how of healthy eating. When you gradually introduce new food items, you ease into new habits without upsetting your usual routine. Soon you'll be eating nutritious food and enjoying it. If you were experiencing breast pain or tenderness, you may notice that it's greatly reduced or gone. Your energy level will increase and your risk of breast infections, cysts, and cancer will be reduced significantly.

This step is also about improving your nutritional intake if you are undergoing treatment for breast cancer. Good nutrition is critical in such cases, because your body is under a great deal of stress and your immune system is compromised.

Step 2: Using Natural Supplements
and Remedies for Healthy Breasts

In today's toxic world, even the best diet needs a boost. If your diet is poor, you need even more help. Nature's bounty can provide the assistance you need. Nutritional supplements, herbal formulas, and homeopathic remedies (such as calcium, calendula, and pulsatilla) can promote, maintain, and restore breast health. Step 2 is about adding natural helpers to your daily routine: something as easy as taking a supplement with breakfast and dinner or enjoying a cup of herbal tea. These simple actions can make a significant difference in your health.

This step also helps women who have breast discomfort or pain, or who are undergoing treatment for breast cancer. Many of Nature's compounds offer healing and restorative powers. Women who are enduring chemotherapy or radiation for breast cancer, or who are dealing with benign breast conditions, will find natural solutions as part of this step.

Step 3: Deciding If Hormones Are Right for You

The decision of whether to take any type of hormone that can affect your health, and especially increase your risk of cancer, is one most women do not take lightly. Nearly every woman has or will face this decision during her lifetime. The great amount of information available, plus what has yet to be discovered, and the fact that each woman has a unique history and set of needs, make it a difficult choice. This step offers you information on the various options when it comes to birth-control pills, hormone replacement therapy, and fertility drugs, and guidelines on how you can make such decisions based on your physical and emotional states.

Step 4: Caring for Your Mind/Body

Understanding the mind/body connection is critical for health and healing. Step 4 includes ways for you to make and keep that connection through exercise, stress reduction, and detoxification. All three are intricately tied together: Exercise heals the body, mind, and soul, reduces stress, and helps detoxify the body. Stress-reduction techniques—guided imagery, meditation, and yoga—relax the body, open up communication between the mind and the body, and aid in the detoxification process. Detoxification techniques, which include fasting, herbal remedies, and manual lymphatic drainage, rid the body of toxins and clear the mind.

Have fun with this step by establishing an exercise routine with friends and learning yoga or meditation. When it comes to detoxification, you may start with herbal remedies or opt for a periodic fast once you discover how good it makes you feel.

Once again, this step includes something for women with breast cancer and benign breast conditions. Suggested exercises for women who have undergone breast surgery are included, and the stress reduction techniques address breast pain, breast cancer, and stress relief.

Step 5: Breast Screening and Preventive Maintenance

Step 5 has three parts: breast self-examination (BSE), examination by a health professional, and mammography. BSE can be done in your own home in a mere 10 to 15 minutes a month, and this step shows you how. Examination of your breasts by a health professional is part of your annual visit to your gynecologist. When you reach the age at which a mammogram is recommended, this quick procedure can be part of your gynecological visit as well, or you can schedule it separately. But perhaps you would rather forego mammography for another screening method. This step explains your options.

You don't have to do all the steps at once, and it doesn't matter in which order you tackle them. But start somewhere, and start today. They could be the healthiest steps you've ever taken.

CHAPTER FOUR

Step 1: Eating for Healthy Breasts

Here's some good news: Between 30 and 50% of all breast cancer could be prevented if people ate a healthy diet and got regular exercise. This important finding by the American Institute for Cancer Research, reached after extensive research analyzed by experts from around the world, is similar to what you'll find in the federal government's National Cancer Institute report, which estimates that one-third of all cancers are related to diet.

Why is this good news? Because it means that you have the power, every time you eat or drink, to maintain and improve your health. Of all the opportunities you have to make choices about your breast health, choosing to fuel your body with life-enhancing natural foods is perhaps one of the most important ones. We are talking about real food—not supplements, herbs, or drugs. Natural, whole food is still the best way for the body to get all the nutrition it needs.

This chapter helps you personally commit to honor and treat your body to nutritious food. It explores healthy food choices for breast health, especially the prevention of breast cancer. It focuses on the latest information from the American Institute for Cancer Research's (AICR) Program for Cancer Prevention, a global research project conducted by the institute along with the World Cancer Research Fund. The result of that project was the world's first major international report on the association between diet and cancer. The report, entitled *Food, Nutrition and the Prevention of Cancer: A Global Perspective*, is the culmination of 4 years of work by 15 of the world's leading diet and cancer researchers with input from more than one hundred other experts from around the world. (See the Resources for the address of the AICR to obtain this report.) A sample menu and recipes that incorporate suggestions from the institute's report are provided.

Other breast-healthy dietary plans are discussed as well, including the Gerson diet and the Super Eight Food Groups diet. All three dietary plans have common elements, including an emphasis on whole grains, fruits and vegetables, and soy products. The benefits of each of these food types are explained and suggestions are offered on how you can include them in your diet. This chapter also discusses which foods are best if you are undergoing chemotherapy or radiation.

Healthy Eating, Healthy Breasts

Eating for healthy breasts is easy and delicious. It is not about sacrifice or giving up burgers and ice cream; it's about discovering new foods and new ways to prepare old favorites. It's about having more energy, feeling better about yourself, and having more control over your health. Basically, it's about improving the quality of your life, for the rest of your life.

Make no mistake: No single diet, food, or supplement can guarantee you won't get cancer. But if you eat a combination of foods that have been shown to prevent cancer and promote health, you can reduce your risk by at least one-third, and more if you follow other healthy habits.

Fortunately, there are many different types of cancer-preventive foods available, perhaps more than you dreamed. Chances are you're already eating some of them, but you may not recognize them when you look at the food on your plate. Are there avocados and fresh spinach under that blue cheese dressing? Are vitamin-rich onions hiding under that fried batter? Can you detect protein-rich, low-fat beans swimming in that beef-laden chili? This step will help you gain a new perspective on healthy foods and expand your culinary horizons.

What We Know About Healthy Eating

The Controversy

Although scores of studies have been done, researchers do not have many definitive answers about the role of foods and nutrients in the prevention of cancer. Many nutritional experts believe, however, that a significant number of Nature's compounds, including vitamins, minerals, and phytochemicals, all of which are explained here and in Chapter 5, help fight cancer. But it has been difficult to measure the actions of these substances because there are so many variables to consider when analyzing the impact of foods and nutrients in humans. That's why the information in this chapter has been culled from the latest and most respected sources, including the American Institute for Cancer Research and the American Dietetic Association.

The American Institute for Cancer Research

To make it easy for you to put together your healthy eating plan, here are the recommendations put forth by the American Institute for Cancer Research's Program for Cancer Prevention, which are explained in detail in its report, *Food, Nutrition and the Prevention of Cancer: A Global Perspective*. These recommendations are the foundation upon which the dietary suggestions in this chapter are based. Although you won't see any radical ideas here, they are universal and the result of years of solid research:

- Choose foods that have undergone little or no processing (e.g., avoid canned, freeze-dried, and frozen foods and foods containing chemical preservatives, colorings, and flavorings).

- The majority or all of your food choices should come from the plant kingdom, which includes fruits, vegetables, legumes, rice, soy foods, whole grains, and foods made from whole grains (and not white, bleached flour), such as pasta, breads, and cereals.

- Eat at least five servings of fruits and vegetables every day (see "How Big Is One Serving" for serving sizes).

- Eat at least seven servings of whole grains, legumes, roots, plantains, and tubers every day.

- Avoid red meat. If you do include animal protein, limit it to no more than 3 ounces per day and choose fish or chicken without the skin. Animal protein should be baked, steamed, broiled, or poached; do not add fat when cooking.

- Limit consumption of dairy products (low-fat and no-fat are better, but they may still contain toxins; see Chapter 9) and other fatty foods. The healthiest oils are olive, flaxseed, and nut. These vegetable oils should be used in moderation and never heated.

- If you drink alcohol, limit your intake to one drink per day.

Armed with this basic outline, along with the warning to avoid sugar and caffeine, you are now ready to look at these foods and the healthy substances they contain.

HOW BIG IS ONE SERVING?

Fruits and Vegetables

1 cup raw leafy vegetables

½ cup cooked or chopped raw fruit or vegetable

1 medium piece of fruit

6 oz. fruit or vegetable juice

¼ cup dried fruit

Grains

1 oz. dry cereal

½ cup cooked rice, grains, pasta

½ English muffin or bagel

3 to 4 plain crackers

1 slice bread

Protein

2 oz. soy-based meat substitute

1½ oz. tofu

2 tbsp. nut butter

½ cup cooked dried legumes or beans

1 egg

½ cup soy milk

1 cup cow's milk

1½ oz. natural cheese

2 to 3 oz. lean meat, poultry, or fish

1 oz. unsalted seeds or nuts

The Soul of Cancer Prevention: Plant Foods

Plant foods—fruits and vegetables, grains, nuts, seeds, and legumes—are rich sources of antioxidants, phytochemicals, enzymes, vitamins, and minerals, as well as fiber and healthy fats. These categories contain thousands of natural compounds, many of which appear to or have been proven to possess potent cancer-fighting properties. Some of the best cancer-protective foods that contain these natural compounds are listed below. These foods should form the foundation of your shopping list.

For tips on how to choose and use the healthiest fruits and vegetables, see "Choosing Healthy Fruits and Vegetables."

Recommended Cancer-Protective Foods

Apples
Apricots
Asparagus
Avocados
Barley
Beans (dried and fresh)
Bok choy
Broccoli
Brussels sprouts
Cabbage
Cantaloupe
Carrots
Cauliflower
Celery
Collard greens
Currants
Dandelion greens
Eggplant
Figs
Flaxseed
Garlic
Grains (see list in this
    chapter)
Grapefruit
Grapes
Guava
Kale
Kiwi
Lemons
Lentils

Mangoes
Mushrooms
Nuts (raw and dry roasted
    only)
Oats
Onions
Oranges
Papaya
Parsley
Pasta (whole-grain)
Peppers
Potatoes
Pumpkin
Radishes
Rice (brown; no bleached
    white)
Sea vegetables
Seeds
Spinach
Squash
Strawberries
Tangerines
Tea (especially green)
Tofu (and other soy-based
    foods)
Tomatoes
Turnips
Watercress
Watermelon

CHOOSING HEALTHY FRUITS AND VEGETABLES

Here are some tips on how to minimize your exposure to pesticides on produce. See Chapter 9 for details about the health hazards of chemically treated foods:

- Buy organic produce and other whole, organic foods, such as grains and nuts. Look for foods that are labeled "certified organic." Organic food offers a nutrition bonus, too. *The Journal of Applied Nutrition* reports that of the organic and conventionally grown produce investigators tested, the organic foods contained 87% higher levels of magnesium, potassium, iron, selenium, boron, chromium, copper, and manganese, and the tomatoes alone had 500% more calcium.

- Scrub fruits and vegetables before eating them. Peel them if they are not organic.

- Eat a wide variety of fruits and vegetables. This minimizes your exposure to any one pesticide.

- If organic produce is too expensive or unavailable, buy organic varieties of the produce that typically contains the highest levels of pesticides and reserve your conventionally grown purchases for produce with less pesticide exposure. Produce highest in pesticide residues include strawberries (worst), cherries, apples, cantaloupe (from Mexico), apricots, grapes (Chile), blackberries, pears, raspberries, nectarines, and spinach. The lowest risk is found in grapes (U.S.), bananas, carrots, green peas, broccoli, cabbage, brussels sprouts, sweet potatoes, cauliflower, onions, corn, and avocados. All other produce falls somewhere in between.

Why Can't I Just Take Supplements?

If these compounds are so potent, why can't you take supplements and achieve the same results? Many experts believe that natural, whole foods are superior to any supplement precisely because they are whole foods—Nature gave each of them a unique combination of phytonutrients that work together to offer specific benefits. Although supplements can play an important part in your program for healthy breasts—and they are discussed in Chapter 5—supplements should be just that: nutrients that add to, or supplement, your basic diet.

Phytochemicals

Switching to a plant-based diet, which is rich in phytochemicals, is one of the most effective cancer-preventive steps you can take (see "Tips for Transitioning to a Healthy Diet," later in this chapter). Phytochemicals are the nonnutrient components of plants that are responsible for giving vegetables, fruits, nuts, legumes, and grains their color, smell, and taste. The American Institute for Cancer Research reports that phytochemicals are exciting because of "their apparent ability to stop a cell's conversion from healthy to cancerous at so many different stages." So far, scientists have identified more than 900 phytochemicals and they are sure more will be discovered.

The American Dietetic Association has identified many phytochemicals that are effective in the treatment and/or prevention of breast and other cancers, heart disease, diabetes, high blood pressure, stroke, and other serious conditions. Below is an explanation of some of the major phytochemicals that have cancer-fighting abilities. Note the foods in which they appear, and then include these foods in your daily plan.

Bioflavonoids

More than 1500 bioflavonoids (also known as flavonoids) have been identified. Because bioflavonoids are found in every plant you consume, eating many different fruits, vegetables, legumes, nuts, and grains will ensure you get a good amount of them. Bioflavonoids are particularly helpful in preventing breast cancer because they detoxify harmful estrogen and inhibit enzymes that produce cancer cells. They also boost the beneficial effects of vitamin C, a powerful antioxidant (see "Antioxidants" in Chapter 5).

Best sources   citrus fruits, red grapes, onions, buckwheat, cruciferous vegetables.

Carotenoids

Several studies have linked carotenoids with a reduced risk of breast cancer, but researchers emphasize that this protection is associated with carotenoids derived from foods and not from supplements. Getting sufficient carotenoids from your diet can be easy, because dozens of foods contain them. Carotenoids are the most common pigments in Nature and are chemically related to vitamin A. In fact, about 50 of them are able to convert into vitamin A in the liver.

BETA-CAROTENE   This is the most commonly recognized carotenoid. Beta-carotene is often called provitamin A because, of all the carotenoids, it is the one most able to convert into vitamin A.

Best sources   beans, carrots, cantaloupe, pumpkin, winter squash, yams, broccoli, brussels sprouts, spinach, sweet potatoes.

Some of the other carotenoids found in foods high in beta-carotene are equally or more responsible for reducing cancer risk. A few of them include lutein, zeaxanthin, lycopene, and canthaxanthin.

LUTEIN AND ZEAXANTHIN   In a study of more than 83,000 women, researchers found that lutein and zeaxanthin provide cancer-fighting benefits for premenopausal women with a positive family history of breast cancer. A National Cancer

Institute study in 1998 also found these two carotenoids to be protective against breast cancer, as well as a third one, lycopene.

Best sources   collard greens, spinach, kale, corn, yellow squash, most yellow fruits and vegetables.

LYCOPENE   This carotenoid is very effective in eliminating the free radicals associated with cigarette smoke (and second-hand smoke) and air pollution.

Best sources   tomatoes and tomato products, carrots, guava, ruby red grapefruit, watermelon. To get the benefits of lycopene in tomatoes, they must ripen on the vine naturally, because lycopene isn't produced until this occurs. Therefore, the tomatoes you buy at the supermarket may have been ripened in transit—off the vine—and may not contain lycopene. Your best bet is to buy organic tomatoes, or grow your own.

Catechins

Catechins also fall into the category of bioflavonoids (see Chapter 5). They hinder the activity of free radicals that are involved in the development of cancer cells.

Best sources   black and green tea.

Chlorophyll

This green pigment prevents damage to the DNA (deoxyribonucleic acid) in cells, which is an initial step in the transformation of normal cells into cancerous ones. All fruits and vegetables contain chlorophyll. Other pigments such as orange, red, and yellow mask chlorophyll in plants of those colors.

Best sources   broccoli, brussels sprouts, kale, parsley, spinach, watercress.

Ellagic Acid

This substance is credited with stopping carcinogens from initiating the cancer cell growth process.

Best sources cherries, grapes, walnuts, raspberries, strawberries.

Genistein

Genistein is believed to be very influential in the prevention of cancer, especially that of the breast and prostate. Because this compound is so important, it is covered in detail later in this chapter (see "The Wonders of Soy").

Best sources soybeans and soy-based foods; also brussels sprouts, cabbage, and collards.

Indoles

The most potent cancer-fighter in this category is indole-3-carbinol. When indole-3-carbinol is taken with the breast cancer drug tamoxifen, it enhances the ability of the drug to prevent the growth of breast cancer cells. This innovative combination may be highly effective in the treatment of breast cancer.

Best sources broccoli, brussels sprouts, cabbage, cauliflower, kale, kohlrabi, mustard greens, rutabaga, savory cabbage, turnips.

Lignans

Lignans not only protect against damage from carcinogens but also help prevent the growth of tumors.

Best sources nuts and seeds, especially flaxseed (see "Using Flaxseed" below).

Limonene

Limonene hinders the ability of cancer cells to use protein, which is necessary for their growth. Studies in which rats with mammary cancer were given limonene show that 80% of the tumors disappeared.

Best sources organic lemon and orange peels, celery seed, mint, dill, and caraway. Use these herbs and seasonings liberally when cooking.

Monoterpenes

These substances stimulate the enzymes that detoxify carcinogens in the body and also act as antioxidants.

Best sources   broccoli, cabbage, carrots, eggplant, fruit, parsley, peppers, squash, tomatoes, yams.

Phenols

Phenols neutralize carcinogens, stimulate the production of detoxifying substances in the body, and limit the damage of free radicals.

Best sources   green tea, garlic, nuts, potatoes, fruit.

Phytosterols

Phytosterols appear to stop the development of breast tumors.

Best sources   the seeds of yellow and green vegetables, although the flesh also has a significant amount.

Protease Inhibitors

These cancer-fighting substances neutralize the effects of certain carcinogens, such as diesel exhaust and radiation.

Best sources   potatoes, soybeans, rice.

Sulforaphane

Sulforaphane helps the body manufacture enzymes that detoxify it of substances such as exhaust fumes and pesticides. It also works along with another detoxifier, glutathione.

Best sources   broccoli, broccoli sprouts, brussels sprouts, cabbage, cauliflower, radishes, rutabaga, and other cruciferous foods.

Fats

Fat has gotten a bad rap. In truth, there are both good and bad types of fat. Everyone needs some fat in their diet to keep the body and brain functioning properly, but it should be healthy, protective fat, such as that found in nuts, avocados, fatty fish, and flaxseed and olive oils.

A role for bad fats in breast cancer seems clear (see Chapter 10). So the overall message about fat is that you need to balance your fat intake—reduce bad fats and increase good fats—while keeping total fat consumption down. Harmful fats are covered in chapter 9; here you will learn about the good fats and how to incorporate them into your diet.

Omega-3 Fatty Acids

Of the various polyunsaturated fats (see Chapter 9), the one that protects against breast cancer, heart disease, arthritis, and psoriasis, is omega-3. It is an essential fatty acid, which means the body needs it to function at its best, and because the body cannot manufacture omega-3, you must get it from your diet.

Omega-3 fatty acids come in three forms: two are found in fish (docosahexaenoic acid [DHA] and eicosapentoaenoic acid [EPA]) and one in plants, especially flaxseed. Several studies have found a link between consumption of omega-3 in the form of cold-water fish and lower rates of breast cancer. Overall, the higher the intake of fish and fish oil, the lower the cancer rates. Conversely, the more animal fat (saturated fat) people eat, the higher the cancer rates.

Other studies support this finding. In 1998, the European Community Multicenter Study on Antioxidants, Myocardial Infarction, and Cancer (EURAMIC) showed that the risk of breast cancer is reduced when the ratio of omega-3 to omega-6 fatty acids (another fatty acid) is increased in fat tissue. Finnish scientists discovered that the breast tissue of women with breast cancer had much lower levels of EPA and DHA than the tissue of women with benign breast disease.

How Omega-3 Fights Cancer

High intake of omega-6 fatty acids can increase the risk of cancer, and high intake of omega-3 fatty acids can protect against it. Omega-6 is not all bad, however, so don't eliminate it altogether. What's important is the ratio of omega-3 to omega-6.

Omega-3 protects against cancer by inhibiting the formation of prostaglandins, which are hormone-like chemicals in the body that are responsible for many functions. Prostaglandin E-2 (PGE-2) is associated with tumor growth and suppression of the immune system's ability to identify tumors. When you consume omega-3 fatty acids as EPA and DHA, they transform into a good prostaglandin, PGE-3, which hinders the production of PGE-2.

Plant Sources of Omega-3

If you don't care for fish or fish oil, or if you are opposed to eating fish, you can get omega-3 from flaxseed, hempseed, peanut, walnut, or other nut oils. Of all these oils, flaxseed is the most concentrated source of linolenic acid and the more common. Refrigerate these oils in a dark jar because they can turn rancid. You can also get DHA from plankton; take as a supplement with food, 100 milligrams three times daily.

Using Flaxseed

Many well-respected physicians, including Michael Murray (*Encyclopedia of Natural Medicine* and other books), Andrew Weil (*Natural Health, Natural Medicine; Eight Weeks to Optimum Health*), Julian Whitaker (*Dr. Whitaker's Guide to Natural Healing*), and Mitchell Gaynor and Jerry Hickey (*Dr. Gaynor's Cancer Prevention Program*), recommend taking 1 tablespoon of flaxseed oil daily, either straight or drizzled on food. You can also add the ground seeds to beverages and food.

To use flaxseeds, grind 2 tablespoons in a coffee or nut grinder. Unground seeds will pass through the body intact and not provide any benefits. Soak the ground seeds in filtered water for 20 minutes to help make the seeds digestible. Add the soaked seeds to juices, health shakes, or food.

Another tasty way to use flaxseed oil is to make a vinaigrette dressing for salads or vegetables. Use both the oil and the soaked seeds, as the latter contain lignans, a type of fiber that has anticancer properties. See the recipe on page 80.

To retain its health-giving properties, refrigerate flaxseed oil in a dark glass bottle and use it within 2 months, or freeze it for up to 1 year. Never heat flaxseed oil. According to Dr. Whitaker, flaxseed oil is very susceptible to damage by light and heat. "Once damaged, the oil is a rich source of toxic molecules known as lipid peroxides. These molecules can actually do the body harm and should not be ingested."

Monounsaturated Fats

The most popular monounsaturated fat is olive oil. High intake of olive oil is associated with a significant decline in breast cancer. Olive oil is very popular among Mediterranean countries, such as Greece, Spain, and Italy, where many studies have been done. These studies reveal a reduced incidence of breast cancer among women who consumed the most olive oil.

In Sweden, the fat intake of more than 61,000 women was analyzed for its association with breast cancer. The investigators found that polyunsaturated fats posed a risk for breast cancer but that monounsaturated fats "might be protective."

Although olive oil is a healthy fat, it loses some of its antioxidant properties if heated at high temperatures and some experts say it may become a carcinogen at very high temperatures. Therefore, do not use olive oil to fry foods. Add it to recipes about a minute before you remove the item from the heat, or drizzle it over prepared foods.

TIPS FOR LOW-FAT EATING

- Use olive oil, flaxseed oil, hemp oil, or nut oils (walnut, almond, macadamia), but do not use over heat or for frying. Suggestions on ways to use olive oil include salad dressings; tossing it with cooked pasta, garlic, and herbs; or to make garlic bread. It is best to avoid fried foods.

- Avoid or greatly eliminate foods containing saturated fats: meat, poultry, and dairy products. If you do eat dairy products, have no more than one serving per day of a low- or no-fat product. Substitute plant-based foods, such as those listed in the "Recommended Cancer-Protective Foods" and "Fiber Content of Common Foods" in this chapter.

- Avoid coconut oil, palm kernel oil, vegetable shortening, and trans-fatty acids (look for the words *hydrogenated* or *partially hydrogenated* on the label). These are found in baked goods, margarine, crackers, and junk foods.

- Try substitutions: Instead of margarine or butter on bread, use olive oil or nut butters. On baked potatoes, use olive oil, salsa, or puréed vegetables with olive oil. In cream soups, use low- or no-fat soy milk. Use nutritional yeast or herb seasoning on air-popped popcorn instead of butter.

Fiber

If you ask most people what fiber is and what it does, you're likely to get some vague answers: "It's in oatmeal, isn't it?" "It cleans out your colon." "Bran muffins have lots of fiber, right?" And if you were to ask about the connection between fiber and breast cancer, you'd probably get some blank stares. But such a relationship exists, and the evidence is clear.

You should know a little about fiber. The human body doesn't have the proper enzymes to digest plant fiber, and there are very good reasons for this fact:

- Fiber absorbs water, which allows stools to pass easily through the intestinal tract.
- Fiber attaches to certain carcinogens and eliminates them from the body.
- Fiber regulates blood sugar levels, which helps people who have diabetes.
- Fiber eliminates cholesterol from the body, which helps keep cholesterol levels down.

Of the two main types of fiber—water soluble (dissolves in water) and insoluble—a controversy exists over which type better protects against breast cancer. For now, both kinds appear to have protective qualities. Examples of foods that contain water-soluble fiber include apples, beans, carrots, citrus fruits, flaxmeal, oats, and oat bran. Some foods with insoluble fiber include celery, corn bran, wheat bran, and the skins of root vegetables and fruits.

The Proof Is in the Fiber

Proof that consuming at least 30 grams of dietary fiber daily can reduce the risk of breast cancer comes from studies around the globe. In Uruguay, scientists found a "strong reduction in risk of breast cancer" related to consumption of a large amount of dietary fiber. An Italian study had the same finding, and noted that premenopausal women seemed to be better protected by fiber intake than postmenopausal women. In France, a 4-year study found that an increase in the amount of fiber, garlic, and onions reduced breast cancer risk. This same study also supported previous reports that saturated fat is a significant risk factor for breast cancer in postmenopausal women.

How Fiber Helps Prevent Breast Cancer

FIBER CONTENT OF COMMON FOODS		
Fiber One cereal	½ cup	10 grams
Prunes (cooked)	½ cup	10
Lentils (cooked)	½ cup	9
Kidney beans (cooked)	½ cup	8
Broccoli (cooked)	½ cup	7
Whole-wheat pita	1	7
Corn	½ cup	5
Whole-wheat pasta	1 cup	5
Chickpeas (canned)	½ cup	5

Lima beans (cooked)	½ cup	5
Apple (with skin)	1 med	4
Peas (cooked)	½ cup	4
Sauerkraut (canned)	½ cup	4
Orange	1 med	4
Strawberries	1 cup	3
Spinach (cooked)	½ cup	3
Cauliflower (cooked)	½ cup	3
Brown rice	½ cup	2
Brussels sprouts	½ cup	2
Zucchini (cooked)	½ cup	2
Carrots (cooked)	½ cup	2

Fiber protects the breasts in several ways:

- Most high-fiber fruits and vegetables also contain a significant amount of isoflavones. These phytoestrogens compete with the body's natural estrogen for estrogen receptor sites (see "The Wonders of Soy" below).
- A high-fiber diet helps eliminate estrogen by binding with it and excreting it.
- High-fiber diets are typically low in fat, which appears to help prevent breast cancer.
- Generally, people who eat a high-fiber diet have lower amounts of body fat and lower levels of estradiol, the most carcinogenic form of estrogen. In contrast, individuals who eat low-fiber, high-fat diets tend to have more body fat, which allows more estrogen to be stored, and therefore increases the risk of breast cancer.

Adding Fiber to Your Diet

The National Cancer Institute recommends that Americans eat 20 to 30 grams of fiber daily, but most of us get only about

11 grams. You can easily increase your fiber intake by adding more fruits, vegetables, and whole grains to your diet and reducing or eliminating meat, dairy, and foods made of white flour and sugar (see "Fiber Content of Common Foods" on pages 61–62). Add fiber gradually. You may experience some gas or stomach discomfort for a week or more as your body adjusts to the increased fiber, but it is temporary.

The Wonders of Soy

The words *soybean* and *tofu* (which is made from soybeans) are misunderstood by many people. Soybeans taste good; some convincing information and ideas are found later in this chapter. Soybeans are also an excellent source of cancer-fighting phytochemicals. Many studies indicate this is true:

- A dramatic indication of the power of soy to prevent cancer is shown in the Japanese diet. The Japanese eat 30 to 50 times more soy products than do Americans. The breast cancer rate among Americans is nearly four times that of the Japanese.

- Studies in animals show that soy, and genistein in particular, inhibits the creation of mammary tumors. In one study, growth of mammary tumors in female rats slowed when they were given soy milk rather than cow's milk.

- At Tufts University School of Medicine, researchers showed that genistein (from soybeans) and curcumin (from turmeric) inhibit the growth of human breast cancer cells induced by pesticides. The authors of the study note that "Since it is difficult to remove pesticides completely from the environment or the diet and since both turmeric and soybeans are not toxic to humans, their inclusion in the diet in order to prevent hormone related cancers deserves consideration."

How Soy Helps Prevent Cancer

Soybeans, which are among the richest sources of plant protein, contain phytochemical substances called isoflavones.
Within this category of biologically active compounds are
several that scientists find have cancer-fighting and cancer-
prevention abilities. Of the three most common of these substances—genistein, diadzen, and glycitein—genistein appears
to be the most powerful cancer fighter, and here's why.

Cancer cells need a reliable blood supply in order to grow
and spread. To ensure such a supply, cancers cells make use of
a process called *angiogenesis*, which is the creation of new blood
vessels. Without a blood supply, cancer cells and tumors stop
growing and can eventually die. Cancer researchers want an
agent that stops angiogenesis. Soy may be that agent.

Researchers are accumulating evidence that soybeans, and
genistein in particular, can help prevent the development of
new blood vessels. A recent study shows that "genistein is a
potent inhibitor of cell proliferation and in vitro angiogenesis." The researchers believe that "these phytoestrogens may
contribute to the preventive effect of a plant-based diet on
chronic diseases, including solid tumors."

Genistein also suppresses the production of stress proteins,
which act as bodyguards to cancer cells. Once genistein
removes these guard cells, the body's immune system can better fight the cancer.

Soy and Its Phytoestrogen Powers

Soy also falls into a category of substances known as phytoestrogens, or plant estrogens. The soybean contains several
phytoestrogens, including genistein and diadzen. These phytoestrogens are similar to the female sex hormone estrogen;
only they are about one thousand times weaker.

Without getting into a detailed discussion of breast cancer
(see Chapter 10), you should know that high levels of estrogen
are related to an increased risk of breast cancer. The breasts

have many estrogen receptors, ready to attract circulating estrogen. But if the much weaker phytoestrogens attach themselves to these receptors, the much stronger estrogen will move on. Thus, scientists believe phytoestrogens, in the form of soy products, help prevent breast cancer, as well as other cancers. The more years a woman eats a diet that is high in soy products, the less exposure her breasts have to estrogen, and the better are her chances of staying breast cancer–free.

Recent studies strengthen the argument that soy products and genistein are effective cancer preventives. At Tufts University School of Medicine in Boston, scientists looked at the damaging effects of environmental chemicals and pesticides and their tendency to stimulate the growth of estrogen receptor–positive breast cancer cells. (See Chapter 10 for an explanation of estrogen receptor–positive cells.) To prevent such growth, the researchers evaluated the effects of curcumin and isoflavonoids on estrogen receptor–positive and estrogen receptor–negative breast cancer cells whose growth was stimulated by the pesticide DDT (chlorophenothane) and other environmental pollutants. They found that the combination of curcumin and isoflavonoids "is the most potent inhibitor against the growth of human breast tumor cells."

Shortly after that study was published, investigators at Wayne State University School of Medicine in Detroit, Michigan, demonstrated how genistein inhibits the growth of specific breast cancer cells, may prevent the spread of breast cancer cells, and promotes a process of cell disintegration known as apoptosis, which appears to be important in limiting tumor growth.

These findings and others support the recommendation to increase the amount of soy in your diet to help prevent breast cancer. Adding soy to your diet can be easy, as you'll see below.

How to Enjoy Soy

All too often, when people think of soybeans they think of tofu, and the classic response is something like "Tofu? I won't eat that stuff." But you can get the benefits of soybeans in many other forms, some so familiar you'll swear you're not eating beans. Soy product manufacturers in recent years have made tremendous advances in improving the taste and texture of soy-based products, such as soy dogs, veggie burgers, and other meat analogues. Items such as chocolate soy shakes, blueberry muffins made with soy flour, and bean chili with tofu are moving into the mainstream. Try adding the following soy products to your daily menu:

- *Soy milk:* Available in plain, vanilla, chocolate, carob, and strawberry. Many varieties are calcium enriched, giving you just as much calcium as cow's milk. Great on cereal and in puddings, milk shakes, sauces, and soups.

- *Soy flour:* Soy flour is made from ground-roasted soybeans and can be used along with other flours when making breads and other baked products.

- *Tofu:* Made from the curd of soy milk, tofu comes in silken, soft, firm, and extra-firm varieties. Use the silken form in puddings, sauces, and protein drinks. The other forms are used to make burgers and meatless loaves or are added to soups, salads, casseroles, and stir-fry. It can be baked or barbequed, marinated or simmered, and it readily absorbs the flavors of the liquid or seasonings in which it is cooked. Think of tofu as you would pasta: Plain spaghetti has little flavor. But when you add sauce, olive oil, and herbs, you have a tasty meal. Tofu is also available prebaked and sea-soned for use as a sandwich filling or snack.

- *Soy yogurt:* Most health food stores carry soy yogurt, which is made with soy milk and bacterial cultures. This excellent substitute for dairy yogurt comes in various flavors.

- *Soybean substitutes for meat and cheese:* They are becoming widely available in mainstream grocery stores. Choose from soy dogs, tempeh (a fermented soy product), burgers, sausage, chicken, beef, pepperoni, and other flavors of animal-product substitutes. These alternatives are low in fat, high in protein, without cholesterol, and good for breast health. You may see the words texturized vegetable protein (TVP) on the labels of some of these products. TVP is also available in raw form, as dried chunks, granules, or flakes. When rehydrated, TVP can be used to make stews, casseroles, soups, sloppy joes, chili, and other dishes.

- *Soy protein extracts:* These liquid forms of soy are a convenient way to add healthy isoflavones to your diet. Just add the amount recommended on the label to juices, milk shakes, or homemade baked goods. Many energy bars contain soy protein extracts.

- *Miso:* Perhaps you've enjoyed miso soup at a Japanese restaurant. If so, you ate a flavored soy paste fermented with salt and rice. Miso is most often used in soups and salad dressings. It contains zybilcolin, which helps eliminate toxins such as nicotine and radiation from the body. Because miso is a live food (contains live enzymes), do not boil it. Add it to your soup or other recipe a minute before you remove the item from the heat.

- *Natto:* This fermented soybean product can be used to make a spread or chutney. It is usually found in the frozen food section of health food or Asian markets.

Other advantages of soy products are that they are high in protein, contain no cholesterol, are usually low in fat, and are rich in isoflavones. Soybeans also contain vitamin K, which helps the blood to clot. If you are taking the anticoagulant drug warfarin (Coumadin), consult with your physician before you add soy products to your diet. Although soy sauce is probably the most recognized of the soybean products, unfortunately the isoflavones are processed out of it. This is not a good source of soy. Plus it is high in salt unless you use the low-salt variety.

Grains, Legumes, and Other Healthy Choices

The American Institute of Cancer Research says a cancer-preventive diet is built on a foundation of seven or more servings per day of grains, cereals, legumes, plantains, and tubers. The options in this category are nearly endless, especially as more and more whole-food manufacturers introduce new products to the market. Take a look at the variety you can add to your breast-healthy diet.

Grains and Cereals

Grains and cereals are the mainstay of diets around the world. Unfortunately, most American grains, cereals, pastas, and rice are overprocessed, leaving behind a pale (literally) reminder of what was once a healthy, whole food. We've been conditioned to believe "white is right" and "down with brown" when it comes to choosing flour, pastas, breads, and rice.

Yet whole grains and the foods made from them are clearly nutritionally superior. Take, for example, whole-wheat flour and enriched white flour. One cup of whole-wheat flour contains more than three times the amount of fiber (about 12 grams) compared with white flour ($3\frac{1}{2}$ grams); more than twice as much calcium, folic acid, vitamin B_5, and zinc; three times as much magnesium, and four times as much phosphorus. All of this goodness originates in whole grains yet, as you can see, much of the nutritional value is stripped away during processing.

Choosing Grains and Legumes

Choose whole, unprocessed products whenever possible. Some grains and grain products say they are "enriched," but this simply means that nutrients have been sprayed on. Most of these added nutrients are easily lost if the grains are cooked in excessive water or rinsed, as is often done with rice and pasta.

AMARANTH is a pale yellow grain that is high in protein and has more calcium than any other grain. It can be used in salads or as a side dish.

BARLEY is often used in salads, soups, pilafs, and as a hot cereal. The pearled barley has been stripped of its nutritional value, so use hulled barley, which still has the bran intact as well as iron, calcium, and phosphorus.

BUCKWHEAT is not really a wheat, and technically it's not a grain either, although it is usually listed as such. It is used in pancakes and breads.

CORN is an all-time favorite that comes in many forms, including polenta, grits, corn pastas, hominy, popcorn, sweet corn, and masa harina (used to make corn chips and tortillas).

KAMUT is used in cold grain salads and as a hot or cold cereal. It is high in protein and minerals.

MILLET is used in casseroles, soups, stews, muffins, and as a cereal. It is a good source of protein, B vitamins, and iron.

OATS, a breakfast favorite, are available as oat bran, oat groats, quick oats, and rolled oats and are a good source of calcium, iron, vitamin E, and most B vitamins.

QUINOA is a complete protein and has the highest protein content of all the grains. It is also a good source of iron, zinc, copper, magnesium, and riboflavin. Use it in stuffing, breads, soups, and stews.

RICE comes in dozens of varieties, but the most common are white, brown, arborio, basmati, jasmine, Texmati, and wehani. Rice is a good source of fiber, B vitamins, iron, magnesium, and phosphorus.

RYE is vastly underused in the United States. It has more protein than whole wheat, and also contains iron and B vitamins. Mix whole rye flour with other whole flours when baking.

TRITICALE is the result of crossing rye and wheat. Triticale is available as flakes, flour, or whole berries. Use it as a cereal or in salads and casseroles.

WHEAT is perhaps the most versatile of all the grains. Whole-wheat pasta and breads are readily available. Also try wheat berries (as a cereal or side dish), bulgur (to make tabbouleh), couscous (as a side dish served like rice), or as the high-protein meat substitute called seitan.

Legumes

This category, which includes beans, lentils, and peas, has been around for at least 10,000 years. Although they've been dubbed the "poor person's protein," they more rightfully should be called the "smart person's protein." Compared with high-fat, high-cholesterol, no-fiber, no-phytochemical meat products, legumes are high protein, high fiber, and full of vitamins, minerals, and cancer-fighting phytochemicals.

Enjoy legumes alone or in soups, stews, casseroles, and chili, made into spreads, or mixed with pasta, grains, or vegetables. They are easy to prepare (see tips below), inexpensive, and store well in airtight containers. The star legume, the soybean, is featured in this chapter.

Roots, Tubers, and Plantains

This category includes vegetables whose primary edible portion is below the ground, such as potatoes, yams, carrots, turnips, beets, rutabaga, parsnips, and kohlrabi. Plantains are a fruit of the tropical perennial herb *Musa paradisiaca* and are a good source of calcium, protein, and phosphorus. They are used as a substitute for potatoes and can be baked or roasted.

Tips for Transitioning to a Healthy Diet

If you are not already eating a plant-based diet, make the transition easily and conveniently with the help of the tips and recipes that follow. Everyone makes changes at a different pace. The secret is to do it gradually but consistently, adding a new food to your diet each day rather than changing every meal. Share ideas with others who are eating healthy. Take a cooking class. Borrow cookbooks from the library or look up vegetarian recipes on the Internet: there are thousands from which to choose. Afraid to try something new by yourself? Experiment with recipes with a friend or ask your kids to help you. Look at your new eating style as an adventure.

Begin by reducing the amount of meat, poultry, and dairy products you eat each day. For example, if you usually have cereal with milk for breakfast, use soy or rice milk on your cereal. For lunch, don't pass up hot dogs or burgers—make a soy dog or a veggie burger. If you want chicken for dinner, have half the amount you usually eat, and add another vegetable or grain to your menu. Next time, eliminate the chicken and replace it with pasta with olive oil and herbs, or maybe a protein-rich chili with TVP.

Shopping for Nutritious Food

The great variety of soy- and vegetable-based meat and dairy substitutes available in mainstream supermarkets is making it easy to adopt a healthy diet. If you want something they don't carry, ask the manager. Demand will create supply. When you go to the market, remember these guidelines:

- The simpler the better: avoid processed, packaged foods loaded with chemical additives. Read the labels.
- Buy organic whenever possible. This includes more than fresh produce. Many organic vegetables, fruits, and grain products are available in packages and cans without chemical preservatives.

- Go with a shopping list. Read through this chapter again and jot down foods from the lists of grains and legumes, soy products, cancer-protective foods, and fiber-rich foods. Get menu and recipe ideas from this chapter, and then get scores more from friends, the Internet, and cookbooks.

Substitutes for Caffeine and Sugar Products

If you are a coffee (or tea or cola) drinker and you want to reduce or eliminate your consumption, there are several ways to make the transition easier. Some people experience caffeine-withdrawal headache when they cut down or quit caffeine intake. To help avoid this reaction, mix half regular and half decaffeinated coffee for a few days and gradually make the switch. Try a natural coffee alternative, such as Pero Coffee Substitute, Postum, and Yerba Mate. Take a similar approach for tea and colas: gradually introduce decaffeinated brands and phase out the caffeinated versions. Herbal teas are an excellent substitute for regular tea, and sparkling waters, flavored and plain, are good alternatives to colas and other sodas.

Most of us ignore the recommendation to limit sweets to once or twice a week. But there is a safe, natural alternative to sugar: stevia. This herb has been used around the world for centuries, but particularly in South America, Japan, China, and Korea. Depending on the form used (concentrate, dried, powder), it is up to 300 times sweeter than cane sugar. If you're weight conscious, it's good to know that stevia is virtually calorie-free. See "Products for Breast Health" in the Resources at the end of this book for suppliers.

You can satisfy your sweet tooth in other ways as well. Honey and maple syrup in small amounts, as well as fruit, help curb the desire for sugar. The following methods also work:

- Eat bitter foods, such as escarole, endive, dandelion, arugula, and broccoli rabe.
- Eliminate coffee. Caffeine increases your desire for sugary foods.

- Reduce the amount of carbohydrates in the form of breads and pasta, which will help reduce your desire for sugary carbohydrates.
- Exercise. It helps reduce cravings for sweets.

Easy Food Preparation Tips

When you get home with your groceries, you're almost ready to cook. The menus and recipes that follow will get you started on the road to better eating. Keep these suggestions in mind:

- Invest in a slow cooker or Crock-Pot. These appliances make preparing grains, beans, rice, soups, chili, and other one-pot meals very easy and time-saving.

- Keep your meals simple, especially while this type of eating is new to you. Plan one basic entree and add other simple foods to complement it. A black bean and barley casserole, for example, can be accompanied by a tossed organic greens salad and whole-grain bread. Steamed broccoli with walnuts goes well with a hearty corn chowder, and everyone loves a baked potato topped with salsa alongside a veggie burger on a whole-wheat bun.

- When preparing basic foods, such as brown rice or lentils, make large portions and freeze the leftovers in meal-size containers. Do the same for one-pot meals such as chili, soups, and stews.

- Be willing to try new things and experiment. Take an old favorite and make it healthy. For example, eliminate the beef from a chili recipe and add TVP instead.

- If you're short on time, try whole-grain pita pockets for quick lunches and snacks. Simply stuff leftovers, vegetables, dips, or sliced or mashed fruit into a pita and you're ready to go.

Sample Menus for Better Breast Health
(asterisked recipes appear in this chapter)

Breakfast 1
Scrambled Tofu with Veggies*
Whole-wheat toast or bagel
Green tea or organic apple juice

Breakfast 2
Potato Scramble*
Breakfast Tempeh Strips*
Fresh Fruit Smoothie* or soy milk

Lunch 1
Veggie Chili with TVP*
Spinach salad
Soy milk

Lunch 2
Easy Tofu Tomato Soup*
Whole-grain crackers
Steamed broccoli with flaxseed oil and garlic
Green tea

Dinner 1
Garlic Pasta with Spinach*
Nutty Green Beans*
Brown Rice Pudding*
Herbal tea or filtered water with lemon

Dinner 2
Delightful Dahl with brown rice*
Whole-wheat pita bread
Cabbage Sprout Salad*
Herbal tea

Snacks

Sunny Quinoa*
Dried apricots and raisins
Fresh Fruit Smoothie*
Fresh fruit
Soy yogurt
Air-popped popcorn with nutritional yeast

Recipes

Scrambled Tofu with Veggies

SERVES 2

> 2 tbsp. filtered water
> ¼ cup each: finely chopped onions, mushrooms, and green or red peppers
> ½ cup chopped tomatoes
> ½ tsp. sea salt
> ½ lb. tofu, crumbled
> ½ tsp. turmeric
> Pepper and basil as desired
> 1–2 tsp. flaxseed oil

Heat the water in a skillet over high flame. Saute the onions, mushrooms, peppers, and tomatoes for about 10 minutes, stirring frequently. Season with salt. Add the tofu and add more water if needed. Season with turmeric, pepper, and basil and cook over medium heat for 5 minutes. Remove from heat, garnish with flaxseed oil, and serve.

Fresh Fruit Smoothie

SERVES 1

> 5 oz. silken tofu
> 6 oz. soy milk (plain or vanilla)
> 1 pint strawberries or blueberries (or ½ pint of each)

2 bananas

1 tbsp. flaxseed (optional)

Place all ingredients in a blender and blend at high speed for 2 to 3 minutes.

Breakfast Tempeh Strips
SERVES 1–2

4 oz. tempeh, sliced into thin strips

3 tbsp. brown rice syrup

1 tbsp. soy sauce

1 tbsp. mustard

3–4 tbsp. filtered water

Pepper to taste

Place all ingredients except pepper in a saute pan with water. Cover and simmer over low heat for 6 to 8 minutes, then turn the strips and simmer for an additional 3 to 4 minutes. Add additional water and 1 extra tablespoon of soy sauce if needed. Season with pepper.

Potato Scramble
SERVES 4

2 medium onions, sliced

1 carrot, sliced thin

¼ cup filtered water

4 potatoes, sliced thin

½ lb. mushrooms, sliced

1 tbsp. tamari

Saute the onions and carrots in water for 5 minutes. Add the potatoes and more water if necessary. Mix well. Cover the pot and steam the vegetables for 15 minutes. Stir occasionally. Add the mushrooms and tamari and cook for an additional 5 minutes. Season as desired.

Veggie Chili with TVP

Hints: Soak the beans overnight to reduce cooking time. Or, in a pinch, you can use precooked organic beans. Or, use a slow cooker (Crock-Pot) and cook on high for 6 to 8 hours or on low for 12 to 14 hours. Chili is great leftover.

SERVES 4

> 2 cups dried red kidney beans
>
> 5 cups filtered water
>
> 2 chopped onions
>
> 2 chopped green peppers
>
> ½ lb. sliced mushrooms
>
> 6 cloves garlic, minced
>
> 2 cups tomato sauce
>
> 1 tbsp. chili powder
>
> 2 cups crushed tomatoes
>
> 1 cup TVP chunks

Place beans in a large pot with the water. Bring to a boil, cover, and simmer for 1 hour. Add the remaining ingredients and cook over low heat for 2 additional hours.

Easy Tofu Tomato Soup

SERVES 2

> 1 red onion, chopped
>
> 1 can tomato soup
>
> 8 oz. firm tofu, diced
>
> 1 cup low-fat soy milk
>
> 1 tsp. basil
>
> ½ tsp. red cayenne pepper
>
> ½ tsp. oregano

Add all ingredients except the spices to a soup pot. Bring to a boil, add the spices, then simmer for 5 minutes.

Garlic Pasta with Spinach

SERVES 3–4

½ lb. whole-wheat spaghetti noodles

¼ cup finely chopped onion

½ lb. fresh spinach, chopped

2 cloves garlic, minced

½ cup filtered water

Salt and pepper to taste

½ cup virgin olive oil

½ cup toasted whole-wheat bread crumbs

Prepare the pasta according to package directions. In a large frying pan, steam the onion, spinach, and garlic in water until spinach is limp. Season with salt and pepper. Drain the pasta and add ⅓ cup of the cooking water to the spinach mixture. Pour in the olive oil and cook the mixture for 1 minute. Place the pasta in a large bowl and pour the spinach mixture over it. Top with bread crumbs.

Nutty Green Beans

SERVES 3–4

2 tbsp. filtered water

1 lb. fresh green beans

1 tbsp. soy margarine

1 tbsp. minced garlic

½ cup whole-wheat bread crumbs

¼ cup chopped walnuts

Salt and pepper to taste

In a medium saucepan, heat the water and saute the beans until tender, about 8 minutes. Reduce the heat and add the margarine, coating the beans. Add the garlic and stir well. Then add the bread crumbs, walnuts, and seasoning.

Delightful Dahl

Serve this traditional Indian dish over brown rice, millet, couscous, or barley.

SERVES 5–6

2 cups filtered water

1 cup green lentils

3 medium potatoes, peeled and cut into bite-size pieces

1 medium onion, chopped

1½ tbsp. curry powder (more or less to taste)

1 tsp. ground coriander

½ tsp. turmeric

½ tsp. dried parsley

Salt and pepper to taste

3 tbsp. olive oil

Bring the water to a boil, add the lentils, lower the heat, and simmer covered for 45 minutes or until the water is absorbed. In a separate pot, boil the potatoes until soft. In a small saucepan, saute the onion, curry powder, coriander, turmeric, parsley, salt, and pepper in a small amount of water for 10 minutes over low heat. During the last minute, add the olive oil and stir well. Turn off the heat, combine the cooked lentils, potatoes, and onion mixture.

Cabbage Sprout Salad

SERVES 2–3

1 cup broccoli sprouts

1 cup mung bean sprouts

2 cups shredded red cabbage

1 cup shredded green cabbage

1 cup shredded carrots

Mix all ingredients together in a bowl. Season with the Basic Vinaigrette dressing on the next page.

Basic Vinaigrette (with variations)

SERVES 1–2

Blend together all of the following ingredients:

> 3 tbsp. red wine
>
> 1½ tbsp. extra-virgin olive oil
>
> 1½ tbsp. flaxseed oil
>
> 2 tbsp. water
>
> 2 cloves finely minced garlic
>
> 2 tbsp. finely minced fresh parsley
>
> ½ tsp. sea salt
>
> 2 tbsp. finely ground flaxseeds

This is the basic vinaigrette. Add any one of the following ingredients and shake well: 1 tbsp. Dijon mustard, or 1 tbsp. fresh minced marjoram, or 1 tbsp. fresh minced basil.

Sunny Quinoa

SERVES 3–4

> 3 cups cooked quinoa
>
> 1 cup seedless red grapes, halved
>
> ¼ cup raisins
>
> 1 tbsp. flaxseed
>
> 1 orange, peeled and cut into bite-size pieces
>
> ½ cup chopped walnuts
>
> 3 apricots, chopped

Place all ingredients in a bowl, cover, and chill for at least 1 hour.

Brown Rice Pudding

> ¼ cup chopped almonds
>
> ½ cup raisins
>
> 1 cup filtered water

3 tbsp. organic unroasted sesame tahini

4 cups cooked brown rice

4 cups soy milk (vanilla if desired)

5 tbsp. maple syrup

2 tsp. vanilla flavoring

Preheat the oven to 350°F. Cook almonds and raisins in water for 3 minutes and blend with the tahini. Stir in the rice, soy milk, maple syrup, and vanilla. Bring the entire mixture to a boil, then simmer uncovered for 10 minutes. Place the mixture in a baking dish with a lid and bake for 40 minutes, then remove the lid and bake another 5 minutes. Serve warm or chilled.

Other Cancer-Fighting Eating Plans

There are several other eating plans that are very healthy and cancer-preventive. Some are based on ethnic and cultural traditions; others on scientific research; and now, the best of both worlds, traditional diets have research to back up their success. Women in many other parts of the world have very low incidences of breast cancer, as well as low rates of heart disease and osteoporosis. Research indicates that diet is a primary reason for these low numbers. Explaining each of these diets is beyond the scope of this book. An overview of two of them can be seen in the pyramid figures. Additional information about these traditional diets can be found in "For Further Reading" in the Resources at the back of this book.

Several other cancer-fighting eating plans include unique qualities that may attract you. This information is meant to whet your appetite for additional details, which you can get by checking out "For Further Reading." In addition to the eating plans explained below, you may want to investigate the Block Anticancer Program, macrobiotics, and the Livingston diet.

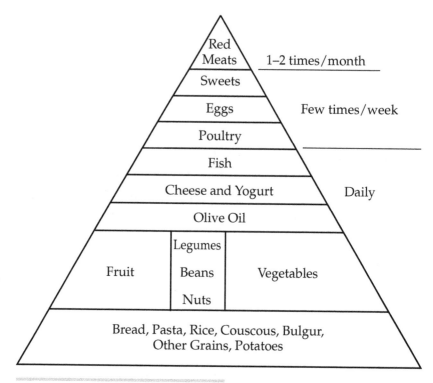

The Mediterranean Diet Pyramid

Gerson Diet Program

The Gerson Diet Program is specially for people with cancer. It combines pure, natural foods and a detoxification program. Max Gerson, M.D., designed the diet after a raw vegetarian diet cured him of migraines. From that point on, he prescribed a raw natural diet for other disorders. He used this approach in his first cancer patient in 1929 and continued to perfect the program. His approach is based on the idea that cancer is the result of faulty metabolism due to poor nutrition and long-term exposure to environmental toxins. To combat these cancer-causing factors and restore the body's natural immunity and healing powers, he recommended organically grown fruits and vegetables, complex carbohydrates, and a strict detoxification program.

To get the maximum benefit from these foods, Gerson prescribed drinking at least 12 glasses of raw juices every day, one

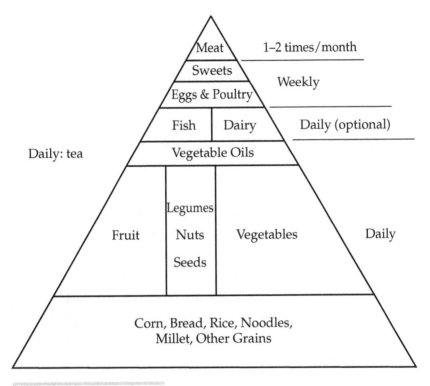

The Asian Diet Pyramid

glass per hour. Different juices are rotated throughout the day. For example, you may start the day with orange juice, then have a mixture of green pepper, lettuce, escarole, watercress, and red cabbage, followed later by a blend of orange, carrot, and celery. Salt use is restricted, because Dr. Gerson believed that excess salt robs the body of potassium, which triggers an imbalance that may lead to cancer.

Part of Gerson's detoxification process involves daily coffee enemas. Gerson believed these enemas eliminate the toxins that are released from dying cancer cells. Coffee enemas stimulate blood flow to the liver, which is the primary filtering organ in the body. Patients also take supplements of linseed oil (rich in omega-3 fatty acids), niacin, and thyroid extract.

The Gerson Diet Program is listed below. Many experts are skeptical about the program, and little research has been done to validate it. One study by cancer researchers in Austria found that individuals on a Gerson-like diet lived an average of 1 year longer than patients not on the plan. Some Gerson patients claim the program has saved their lives.

GERSON DIET PROGRAM

Allowed: Fruits, whole vegetables, salad vegetables, juices of fruits, vegetables and leaves, potatoes, oatmeal, bread, whole grains.

Forbidden: Salt, salt substitutes, and salty foods; all processed foods (canned, frozen, jarred, boxed); smoked food, sulfured food, fats, nuts, and oils; meat and fish; dairy products (allowed in small amounts for some individuals, but only after several months of treatment); alcohol; spices; cake, candy, and other sugary foods; vegetables high in sodium; drinking water (the Gerson Diet provides a high volume of water from fruits and vegetables, especially the juices).

Super Eight Food Groups Diet

An eating approach developed by J. Robert Hatherill, Ph.D., author of *Eat to Beat Cancer*, is based on years of intense research. Dr. Hatherill's approach, which he says can help people avoid up to 90% of all cancers, is based on eight food groups. Each plant-based group contains chemopreventive foods that offer unique health benefits not duplicated by the other groups. An explanation of each of the groups and their primary benefits appears below.

SUPER EIGHT FOOD GROUPS

1. *Onion group:* onion, garlic, asparagus, shallots, leeks, chives, scallions. Prevent tumors, inhibit cancer, block formation of cancer-causing substances.

2. *Cruciferous group:* broccoli, cabbage, cauliflower, brussels sprouts, turnips, and others. Contain glucosinolates,

sulfur-containing compounds that have anticancer properties.

3. *Nuts and seeds:* sesame seeds, pumpkin seeds, almonds, walnuts, and others. Contain protease inhibitors, which can reduce incidences of breast cancer.

4. *Grass group:* amaranth, corn, barley, flaxseed, millet, oats, rice, wheat, and others. Contain lignans, which have an antiestrogen effect and suppress the growth of breast cancer.

5. *Legume group:* soybeans (including all soy products), peas, beans. Contain protease inhibitors and genistein. Of all the legumes, soybeans contain the greatest amount of saponins, which are potent chemopreventive substances.

6. *Fruit:* citrus, berries, melons. These fruits increase the activity of the enzyme glutathione-S-transferase (GST), which deactivates carcinogens.

7. *Solanace group:* tomatoes, potatoes, sweet potatoes, beets. Tomatoes are especially helpful because they contain substances that inhibit the formation of carcinogens.

8. *Umbelliferous group:* celery, carrots, dill, anise, fennel, parsnips, cumin, coriander, parsley, celeriac, caraway. This group is rich in plant chemicals called phytochemicals, which have anticancer properties.

Dr. Hatherill emphasizes that "The relatively few vitamins and minerals that exist each have precisely defined nutritional roles. In contrast tens of thousands of potentially important anticancer collages are present in whole foods." In addition to eating from the eight food groups, he recommends using licorice, rosemary, cayenne, tumeric, and green tea. Sea vegetables are encouraged because of their antitumor and antioxidant powers. His plan also includes the following recommendations:

- Avoid burnt or overcooked foods. The best ways to cook are to bake, steam, broil, or microwave.
- Avoid fried foods.
- Take a high-quality multivitamin/mineral, especially vitamins A, C, E, and B$_{12}$, and the mineral selenium.
- If you must cook with oil, use only olive, sesame seed, or macadamia oils.

What to Eat During Cancer Treatment

The foods discussed in this chapter help promote healthy breasts. But certain foods are especially protective if you have breast cancer and are undergoing radiation or chemotherapy. Specific herbs and supplements to help you through these toxic treatments are discussed in Chapter 5. They can be taken along with the dietary suggestions given below.

Diet and Chemotherapy

Chemotherapy places a great deal of stress on a body that is already somewhat compromised. Therefore, you need foods that provide maximum nutrition, low fat, and minimal stress on the liver and digestive system. One to two weeks before you begin chemotherapy, help balance your body with healthy blood sugar levels and low toxicity. You can do this by focusing on the following foods and eating four to six smaller meals a day:

- All vegetables, organic preferred
- Fruits (avoid very sweet ones), organic preferred, especially apples, cherries, grapefruit, papaya, pineapple
- Complex carbohydrates from whole-grain sources: whole-wheat breads and pasta, oatmeal, and any of the grains
- Low-fat protein foods such as soybeans and soy foods, lentils, chickpeas, peas, beans, or cold-water fish

Some foods are best avoided:

- Animal foods (meats, eggs, dairy)
- Simple carbohydrates, especially processed, sugary foods

- Sweet fruit juices and soft drinks
- Alcohol, caffeine, and other stimulating foods
- Spicy foods

These food guidelines can be followed throughout your therapy if you do not experience significant nausea or loss of appetite. If you do have stomach difficulties, eat small, frequent meals of bland, easy-to-digest foods such as mashed potatoes, plain oatmeal or cream of wheat, soy or rice milk, dry whole-wheat crackers or pretzels, vegetable broth, brown rice flavored with vegetable broth, plain soy yogurt, or boiled or baked chicken without the skin.

Diet and Radiation

Foods that strengthen DNA against radiation include those high in carotene, including dark leafy greens, dandelion greens, sweet potatoes, pumpkin, and orange winter squash. Soybeans and tofu, which are good sources of protease inhibitors, guard against radiation damage. Because protease inhibitors are destroyed if these foods are cooked at high temperatures, steam tofu (you can still marinate it first) and roast soybeans. Other foods that offer protection include miso, buckwheat, burdock root, apples (with the skins on, so buy organic), sunflower seeds, flaxseed oil, and lentils.

Experts also recommend that you eat four to six small, low-fat meals daily. Also observe the list of foods to avoid, and drink eight or more glasses of bottled or filtered water per day.

The impact of diet on health is staggering, and in the case of cancer, the evidence is not only impressive but documented in countless studies. That's why Step 1 of the healthy breast program is so important. Every time you have a meal, a snack, or a beverage, you hold in your hands the power to fight cancer and enhance your overall health. Conversely, those same hands can hold damaging foods. The choice is up to you.

CHAPTER FIVE

※

Step 2: Using Natural Supplements and Remedies for Healthy Breasts

Everywhere you turn, you see ads for supplements. If you were to take all the supplements that are touted, you would be popping capsules all day.

So why devote a step for breast health to using natural supplements and remedies? Because often the body needs extra help in the form of vitamins, minerals, and other nutrients, or herbal or homeopathic remedies, to correct a deficiency or facilitate the healing process. Because even though you want to eat nutritious meals, sometimes you're too busy to achieve that goal. Because unless you buy organic or whole foods, much of the food on the market lacks adequate nutritional value. Because there are many things in the environment that deplete nutrients from your body, including physical and emotional stress, pollution, insufficient sleep, smoking, over-the-counter (OTC) and prescription drugs, caffeine, and alcohol. Because sometimes you experience symptoms that respond well to natural remedies, which allows you to avoid use of conventional drugs and their associated side effects. Because you may be under necessary chemotherapy or radiation treatment and your body can benefit from the healing powers of natural remedies.

That's why Step 2 of the Five-Step Program for Breast Health is important. This chapter brings that step to you in three sections. The first explains and gives doses for various vitamins, minerals, and other nutritional supplements you should consider adding to your daily routine to optimize your breast health. The second discusses natural remedies, including supplements, herbs, and homeopathic remedies, for benign breast conditions. The third offers similar natural remedies for women who are undergoing chemotherapy or radiation treatment. Several remedies fit into more than one of these categories, and how you use them may differ, so some remedies appear more than once. Consult with your physician if you are taking any herb or supplement for a breast condition, especially if you are undergoing cancer treatment. Natural, complementary therapies can be powerful, and they may interact with other substances.

Supplements for Overall Breast Health

At minimum, all women need to take a multivitamin-mineral supplement, even those who eat a healthy diet, because of the reasons just mentioned. Think of your supplement as an insurance policy: it's no guarantee that you won't get sick, but it's an economical, safe way to help promote and maintain breast health. The recommended supplement dosages for overall breast health are shown below. To help you understand the importance of these supplements to your breast health, a brief explanation of some of them follows.

RECOMMENDED MULTIVITAMIN-MINERAL FORMULA

Vitamins

Vitamin A (preferably as beta-carotene)	5000 IU
Beta-carotene (if not as vitamin A)	25,000 IU
Vitamin D	400 IU
Vitamin C	500 mg
Vitamin E (mixed natural)	400 IU
Vitamin B_1 (thiamin)	100 mg
Vitamin B_2 (riboflavin)	50 mg
Vitamin B_3 (niacin)/Niacinamide	10 mg/150 mg
Vitamin B_5 (pantothenic acid)	25 mg
Vitamin B_6 (pyridoxine)	25 mg
Vitamin B_7 (biotin)	300 mcg
Folic acid	400 mcg
Choline	100 mg
Inositol	100 mg

Minerals

Boron (chelate)	1 mg
Calcium (citrate)	500 mg*
Chromium	200 mcg
Copper (gluconate)	2 mg
Iodine	150 mcg
Iron	15 mg[†]
Magnesium	500 mg
Manganese (aspartate)	10 mg
Molybdenum (chelate)	100 mcg
Potassium	99 mg
Selenium	200 mg
Vanadium (chelate)	25 mcg
Zinc	20 mg

Bioflavonoids

100 mg

*Take an additional 500 mg calcium supplement. The ratio of calcium to magnesium should be 2:1 (i.e., 1000 mg calcium and 500 mg magnesium). You may take all of your calcium and magnesium as a separate combination supplement if desired.

[†]Postmenopausal women do not need to take iron. Before taking a supplement with iron, ask your doctor to check your iron levels. Iron is very toxic if too much is taken.

Antioxidants

Antioxidants are any vitamin, mineral, or other nutrient that fights or works against (*anti*) the cell-damaging process called *oxidation*. The substances responsible for oxidation are called *free radicals*, molecules that have an unpaired electron in their structure and thus circulate through the body in search of a mate. Unfortunately, free radicals are found in harmful substances, such as cigarette smoke, toxic chemicals, radiation, fried and processed foods, and other pollutants. When these free radicals find other molecules in the body that have an even number of electrons, they steal those electrons, and in the process create more free radicals. This process of free radical damage (oxidation) is associated with more than sixty medical conditions, including cancer.

To fight free radicals, you need antioxidants. Although the best sources of most antioxidants are fresh fruits and vegetables, you can enhance your diet and your breast health by taking supplements. Four of the most common antioxidants (vitamins A, C, and E, and the mineral selenium; known collectively as ACES) are discussed below. They are standard ingredients in multivitamin-mineral supplements. Several other antioxidants that may help prevent breast cancer are covered later in this chapter.

Vitamins A, C, and E

Three of the four antioxidants many experts consider the most important in the fight against cancer in general are vitamins A (as beta-carotene, also classified as a carotenoid; see below), C, and E. These vitamins enhance the immune system to prevent cancer. In the fight against breast cancer in particular, the evidence is less conclusive but growing.

A 1998 Cornell University study noted that the "best evidence" of reduced cancer risk was with vitamins A, D, and E, with "less consistent evidence" for vitamin C. A more recent study published in the *Journal of the National Cancer Institute* evaluated the association between risk of breast cancer and intake of specific carotenoids, vitamins A, C, and E, and fruits and vegetables in more than 83,000 women who participated in the Nurses' Health Study. The researchers concluded that there was a reduced risk of breast cancer in premenopausal women with a family history of breast cancer who had five or more servings per day of beta-carotene and vitamins A and C than those who had only two servings daily.

Selenium

Selenium can help increase the number of white blood cells, which the immune system requires to fight pathogens. It also works with vitamins C and E to eliminate free-radical production. These properties led Dr. Gethard Schrauzer of the University of California, San Diego, to suggest that one reason Utah has the lowest cancer rate in the United States is that its soil has a very high concentration of selenium. And at the University of Arizona, scientists discovered that daily supplementation with selenium decreased the risk of various cancers by up to 60%.

What to Look For

When reading the label of a multivitamin-mineral for its vitamin E content, look for those that say "d-alpha tocopherol." This is the natural form of vitamin E, which is better absorbed by the body than the synthetic form.

Vitamin A is a fat-soluble vitamin, which means the body stores it. Because large amounts of this vitamin can cause significant side effects (such as headache, liver and nerve damage, vomiting, and birth defects), it is best to get your vitamin A through beta-carotene, which does not cause these reactions. Beta-carotene also has cancer- and heart disease–fighting properties that vitamin A does not have. It is safe to get a supplement that has a mixture of both vitamin A and beta-carotene.

Vitamin C is available in several forms, including sodium-L-ascorbate, sodium-D-ascorbate, and ascorbic acid. Avoid the sodium or salt forms if you have high blood pressure.

Some nutritionists say that a natural form of selenium, called L-selenomethionine or selenium-rich yeast, is better utilized by the body than the synthetic forms. So far, no one has proved this to be true.

Vitamins and Minerals

In addition to the antioxidants already mentioned, several other vitamins and minerals have cancer-fighting properties. Notice the many foods that contain these breast-healthy nutrients.

B Vitamins

The B vitamins are considered as a family because they work closely together in metabolic processes and in strengthening the immune system in its fight against cancer. Although each individual B vitamin may not possess specific cancer-fighting powers, collectively they appear to have anticancer abilities.

VITAMIN B_1 (thiamin) works closely with vitamins B_6 and E to eliminate the toxic effects of tobacco smoke and alcohol. Good sources are bulgur, brewer's yeast, brown rice, chickpeas, navy beans, sunflower seeds, wheat germ, and whole-grain flour.

VITAMIN B_2 (riboflavin) plays a key role in the production of the powerful antioxidant glutathione (see below). You'll find vitamin B_2 in broccoli and broccoli sprouts, fortified cereals and breads, spinach, and sweet potatoes.

VITAMIN B_3 (niacin/niacinamide) appears to increase the ability of the cells to resist cancer growth. Good sources are barley, bulgur, brewer's yeast, beets, chicken breast, peanuts, and sunflower seeds.

VITAMIN B_5 (pantothenic acid) helps in the manufacture of red blood cells and enhances the immune system. It is found in corn, green leafy vegetables, lentils, mushrooms, nuts, and whole-grain cereals.

VITAMIN B_6 (pyridoxine) is essential because low levels suppress the immune system. Get vitamin B_6 in avocados, bananas, brown rice, carrots, lentils, soybeans, and whole grains.

FOLIC ACID also known as folate and folacin, appears to inhibit the transformation of normal cells into cancerous ones. Enjoy asparagus, avocado, beans (pinto, adzuki, and black), black-eyed peas, spinach, chicory, romaine lettuce, papaya, and parsley.

VITAMIN B$_{12}$ helps maintain an efficient immune system. Although this vitamin is found primarily in meat and dairy products, many foods are fortified with B$_{12}$, including cereals and soy products. Natural sources of B$_{12}$ are nutritional yeast and sea vegetables, such as kelp, dulse, and other seaweeds.

Calcium

Many women have the misconception that they must consume dairy products to get enough calcium. Yet soybeans, soy products, legumes, beans, cruciferous vegetables, calcium-enriched orange juice, and seaweed provide an excellent supply of calcium, plus you get cancer-fighting phytochemicals and a good dose of protein. One cup of cow's milk, fortified soy milk, and fortified rice milk all contain about 280 milligrams of calcium. Soy products also contain the all-important phytoestrogens, explained in detail in Chapter 4.

Calcium has been identified as a cancer-preventive nutrient. At the Strang Cancer Research Laboratory at Cornell University, scientists found that "decreased calcium and vitamin D intake and high dietary fat are associated with mammary gland carcinogenesis" and there is a "possible role for increased dietary calcium and vitamin D" in the prevention of breast cancer.

Vitamin D

Vitamin D, the "sunshine vitamin"—so named because the body produces it when exposed to the sun for about 10 minutes a day—has been associated with a reduced risk of breast cancer in several studies. In 1999, for example, researchers with a National Health and Nutrition Examination Survey study reported that their "data support the hypothesis that sunlight and dietary vitamin D reduce the risk of breast cancer."

Other Recommended Natural Supplements

In addition to a multivitamin-mineral supplement, several other substances can be a helpful part of your breast health program. They include glutathione, green tea, indoles, red clover, and soy isoflavonoids. You may want to include these as part of your overall breast health program, especially if you are at risk for breast cancer.

In this section and others throughout the chapter you will be directed to take or use an herbal remedy. An explanation of the way herbs can be used appears in "Forms of Herbal Remedies."

FORMS OF HERBAL REMEDIES

Infusion

A strong tea made from the soft parts of an herb, including the leaves and flowers. A typical infusion is made by pouring 1 cup of boiled water over 1 to 2 teaspoons of dried herbs or 3 to 6 teaspoons of fresh herbs. Steep the herbs for 10 to 15 minutes in the covered pot. Strain the infusion and discard the herbs.

Decoction

A decoction involves use of herb parts that have thick cell membranes, including the roots, stems, and bark. Place 1 teaspoon of dried herbs or 1 tablespoon of fresh herbs in a pot and add 8 ounces of cold water. Bring to a boil and allow to simmer, covered, for 5 to 30 minutes, depending on the herb. Strain and discard the herbs.

Extract

An extract is a concentrated combination of powdered herbs with either water or alcohol. Many herbs are available in a standardized form, which is a way to ensure uniform potency. The terms *extract* and *tincture* are often used interchangeably, and for treatment purposes they are similar.

Tincture

A concentrated herbal form composed of either fresh or dried herbs combined with alcohol or glycerine.

Poultice

A thick, warm, herbal paste applied to the skin to treat pain and inflammation. It is usually prepared by adding hot water to dried powdered herbs to create a paste. Once the poultice is applied, it should be covered with a hot, moist towel and remain in place until the mixture cools.

Glutathione

This powerful antioxidant is key in eliminating toxins from the body through the liver. It also protects against free-radical damage and strengthens cell membranes. Some foods are rich in glutathione, such as avocados, raw spinach, asparagus, walnuts, potatoes, pears, watermelon, and apples, while others help stimulate the body's production of this antioxidant. Cruciferous vegetables fulfill both roles. Garlic, chives, onions, and leeks help increase the body's ability to use glutathione.

If you have breast cancer, increasing glutathione levels in your body may be helpful. You can help your body produce more glutathione by eating foods that are rich in the amino acid cysteine, such as beans and whole grains, or you can take a cysteine supplement (see "Cysteine," later in this chapter). To encourage elimination of toxins from the body and to interfere with the production of cancer cells, glutathione also needs calcium (see "Calcium" above).

Green Tea

The freshest, least processed form of tea is green tea (*Camellia sinensis*). Green tea contains high levels of polyphenols, substances that neutralize free radicals associated with cancer, and is a rich source of antioxidants. Green tea protects against breast cancer by preventing initiation of cancer growth. Three to five cups of green tea daily are recommended for cancer prevention. Green tea is available loose, in tea bags, or in capsules. Take according to package directions. Green tea contains caffeine, although you can buy decaffeinated forms.

Indoles

Indoles are a type of phytochemical found in cruciferous vegetables, such as broccoli, cabbage, and cauliflower. Their ability to protect against breast cancer seems to be related to their tendency to inhibit estrogen and to promote the activity of protective enzymes. Researchers at the Strang Cancer Prevention Center in New York City believe they demonstrated this when they studied 60 women at increased risk for breast cancer and gave half of them 300 milligrams daily of indoles and half of them a placebo. They determined that 300 milligrams of indoles per day may be "a promising chemopreventive agent for breast cancer prevention" and encouraged further studies to help identify the most effective dose.

Red Clover

Red clover (*Trifolium pratense*) is a rich source of phytoestrogens, surpassing soybeans in the number of these cancer-fighting compounds that it makes available, especially genistein. This herb also helps cleanse the lymphatic system and bloodstream of toxins (see also "Natural Remedies for Benign Breast Conditions," later in this chapter). To use red clover as an infusion, pour 8 ounces of boiling water over 2 to 3 teaspoons of dried flowers. Cover and steep for 10 to 15 minutes. Drink up to 3 cups per day. If you take the tincture, use 2 to 4 milliliters in water three times a day. Red clover is available either fermented or nonfermented. The nonfermented form is safe and does not cause side effects. Avoid the fermented product.

Soy Isoflavonoids

You read about the importance of soy in Chapter 4. Increase your intake of soy products by taking a soy isoflavonoid supplement. A 500- or 1000-milligram tablet once or twice daily, depending on your intake of soy foods, is recommended. Look for supplements that contain 12 to 20 milligrams of genistein and diadzein per dose.

Side Effects of Radiation and Chemotherapy

Radiation weakens the immune system because it is a carcinogen. Radiation oncologists use a highly focused beam on the tumor to kill cancer cells while trying to minimize the damage to surrounding tissue. Some toxic radiation does extend beyond the tumor site, however, and often causes hair loss, weakness, nausea, and vomiting. Radiation destroys the ability of antibodies to fight infection and cancer and can damage the thymus gland, which produces cancer-fighting T cells.

The drugs used to destroy the cancer cells left behind after surgery are toxic as well. In most cases, two or more cancer-fighting drugs are used in chemotherapy, because it's been shown that combination therapy works better than single drugs. Unfortunately, this mixture can make the side effects worse and make it difficult for the body to absorb the nutrients it needs to keep the immune system operating efficiently.

Natural Remedies During or
After Chemotherapy and Radiation

One major advantage of taking natural substances either during or after cancer treatments is that they enhance the immune system, protect it against the toxic abuses of radiation and chemotherapy, and help eliminate the toxins from the body. Eating foods that are high in the nutrients discussed below is also recommended (see Chapter 4), as well as drinking at least eight glasses of filtered water each day.

The suggested natural remedies explained below complement conventional medical therapies and in no way should replace them. Discuss any natural approach you wish to add to your treatment program with your medical team. Homeopathic remedies (see below) may be helpful and should be taken under the supervision of a homeopath or other health care professional knowledgeable in homeopathy.

HOMEOPATHIC REMEDIES FOR RADIATION AND CHEMOTHERAPY EXPOSURE

To relieve radiation side effects:

- *Cadmium iodatum:* relieves nausea and antidotes radiation poisoning
- *Cadmium sulphuratum:* antidotes radiation poisoning
- *Ferrum metallicum:* treats anemia
- *Ipecac:* relieves nausea
- *Nux vomica:* relieves nausea

To relieve chemotherapy side effects:

- *Cadmium sulphuratum:* relieves nausea
- *Ferrum metallicum:* treats anemia
- *Hydrastis:* relieves stomach distress
- *Ipecac:* relieves nausea
- *Nux vomica:* relieves nausea
- *Opium:* relieves nausea

Multivitamin-Mineral Supplement

Chemotherapy typically causes poor absorption of nutrients, weight loss, nausea, and vomiting, all of which can severely compromise an already weakened immune system. Therefore, a daily high-potency multivitamin-mineral supplement is recommended. Several animal and laboratory studies have indicated that vitamins A, C, and E boost the effectiveness of chemotherapy, although no human studies have been done.

If the supplement you choose does not meet the recommended dosages indicated for selected vitamins and minerals outlined in the section below, you will need to supplement those nutrients separately. If you are taking the chemotherapy drug methotrexate, do not take a multiple supplement that contains more than 400 micrograms of folic acid, because it may interfere with the drug's effectiveness. Some physicians prescribe a special folic acid called leucovorin to help protect against side effects caused by methotrexate.

Astragalus

Researchers at M.D. Anderson Cancer Center in Houston have investigated the use of this herb as an adjunct to cancer therapy. When taken after a course of chemotherapy, astragalus can help the bone marrow produce white blood cells and boost the immune system. The recommended dosage is two to three 500-milligram capsules three times a day.

Beta-carotene

Beta-carotene increases the body's levels of the tumor-fighting proteins called cytokines, as well as cancer-fighting antibodies and natural killer cells. It is a precursor for vitamin A, which means it transforms into a form of vitamin A as the body needs it. Beta-carotene is less toxic than vitamin A and has disease-preventive properties that regular vitamin A does not have.

Take between 15,000 and 30,000 international units of beta-carotene daily (10–20 milligrams). Beta-carotene is available in capsules and tablets and as part of a multivitamin-mineral supplement. Some people develop an orange tinge to their skin if they take more than 50,000 international units daily, but this is harmless and disappears when the dose is lowered.

If you are taking the chemotherapy drug methotrexate, even higher doses of beta-carotene are suggested, because this drug can have a devastating effect on the liver. A daily dose of 50,000 to 75,000 international units (30–50 milligrams) can be taken beginning about 2 weeks before therapy and continuing during therapy.

B Complex Vitamins

The B complex vitamins help raise the number of cancer-fighting white blood cells. Not every B vitamin plays a critical role in fighting cancer, but because all the B vitamins work together, take a B complex and then supplement with additional specific B vitamins if needed.

Vitamin B_6 (pyridoxine) is often needed in higher amounts because it helps reduce the nausea associated with chemotherapy and radiation. Beginning about 2 weeks before treatment and continuing during treatment, take 50 to 100 milligrams daily or up to 150 milligrams daily for a shorter time if nausea is severe. Up to 300 milligrams may be acceptable in cases of severe nausea and vomiting, but only take this dose if you are under the direct care of a nutritional specialist.

Choline

Choline is a coenzyme that is utilized during metabolism. It is produced by the body when vitamin B_{12}, folic acid, and the amino acid methionine work together. As a supplement it can be found in many multivitamin-mineral combinations, or it is found in the supplement lecithin, which is a source of both choline and inositol, a vitamin-like substance. Consider the following guidelines for choline:

- If you take the chemotherapy drug vincristine (Oncovin), supplement with 1000 milligrams of choline daily in the form of soy lecithin granules to help the nervous system. One teaspoon of soy lecithin granules equals approximately 250 milligrams of choline.

- If methotrexate is part of your chemotherapy regimen, take 1000 milligrams of choline beginning 2 weeks before therapy and continuing during therapy.

Coenzyme Q_{10}

The powerful antioxidant coenzyme Q_{10} (CoQ_{10}) (a catalyst that promotes chemical reactions in the body without being destroyed or damaged by the reactions) occurs naturally in the body. Its value in the fight against cancer was first documented by Dr. Karl Folkers, who in the 1930s discovered that his cancer patients who took the antioxidant lived unexpectedly longer than patients not taking the remedy. Since then, it has been found to protect against chemotherapy-induced cardiac toxicity, which is a very common side effect of the drug doxorubicin (Adriamycin). For this reason, some doctors recommend taking 90 to 120 milligrams daily of CoQ_{10}.

A French clinical trial studied 200 women who were suspected of having breast cancer. A deficiency of CoQ_{10} was found in the 80 women who were eventually diagnosed with breast cancer as well as in the 120 women who had nonmalignant lesions. These findings suggest CoQ_{10} may help prevent or fight breast cancer.

Danish researchers administered 90 milligrams of CoQ_{10} on a daily basis, several other antioxidants, and fatty acids to 32 patients with breast cancer. In six patients the tumors regressed partially. When one of the six patients was then given 390 milligrams of CoQ_{10} daily for 2 months, the tumor disappeared. Another patient who had residual tumor after surgery was treated with 300 milligrams of CoQ_{10} daily for 3 months, and that tumor also disappeared. Although nothing definitive can be derived from these cases, some researchers say they support the belief that CoQ_{10} fights breast cancer in at least some women.

Suggested doses of CoQ_{10} for women who have breast cancer are from 90 to 390 milligrams daily. Low doses may reduce pain, increase appetite, and decrease metastases. When 300 to 390 milligrams are given daily, some patients have reported partial or complete remission of their cancer. Coenzyme Q_{10} is available in tablets, capsules, or oil-based gel capsules. Because CoQ_{10} is fat soluble, it is better absorbed when taken with fat.

If you don't use the gel capsules, take the capsules or tablets with a bit of fatty food, such as avocado.

Coenzyme Q_{10} rarely causes side effects. At very high doses (600 milligrams or higher), heartburn, headache, fatigue, diarrhea, and involuntary movements may occur.

Cysteine

If you have breast cancer, include the supplement cysteine in your recovery plan. Look for cysteine in the form of N-acetyl-L-cysteine (NAC) capsules. Take 1800 milligrams per day to help reduce the nausea and vomiting caused by chemotherapy. NAC is also available as an ointment, which can help prevent hair loss and decrease skin burns associated with radiation therapy.

Evening Primrose Oil

Evening primrose (*Oenothera biennis*) seeds contain a high level of gamma-linolenic acid, or omega-6 fatty acids. If you take the chemotherapy drug vincristine (Oncovin), evening primrose oil can enhance its effectiveness. Take one 500-milligram capsule one to three times daily.

Ginger

Ginger can help alleviate nausea and vomiting associated with chemotherapy. Suggested dosages include 2 to 4 grams of dried rhizome powder two to three times a day; or a 250-milligram tablet or capsule every 2 to 3 hours, not to exceed 1 gram daily. Excessive ginger may cause heartburn.

Ginseng

In December 1999, researchers at Harvard Medical School in Boston reported that American ginseng inhibited the growth of human breast cancer cells in the laboratory. In Russia, researchers found that Siberian ginseng helped protect against side effects from radiation therapy. Both Siberian and Asian ginseng have been recommended following chemotherapy. The dosage for Siberian ginseng is 2 to 3 grams per day of the dried root or 300 to 400 milligrams per day of the solid extract standardized on eleutherosides B and E. If taking the Asian form, the suggested dosage is 100 to 200 milligrams per day of the standardized herbal extract.

Ginseng is generally very safe, but it may cause insomnia. Do not use ginseng if you have high blood pressure or if you are pregnant or breast-feeding. Long-term use of ginseng may cause tender breasts and menstrual abnormalities.

Medicinal Mushrooms

According to Andrew Weil, M.D., author of *Natural Health, Natural Medicine: Eight Weeks to Optimum Health*, medicinal mushrooms are recommended if you "are recovering from chronic illness, undergoing cancer treatment . . . or merely want to strengthen your body's defenses." Medicinal mushrooms, which include maitake, shiitake, and reishi, help eliminate toxins from the body because they are a rich source of phytochemicals. Reishi fights tumors and helps produce an antitumor substance called tumor necrosis factor. Reishi is available as a tea, extract, or powder. The recommended daily dose is 3 to 5 grams. Occasionally it may cause dizziness, dry mouth and throat, abdominal upset, and nosebleeds if used continuously for more than 3 months. Do not take reishi if you are taking anticoagulants or if you are pregnant or breast-feeding.

Maitake inhibits tumor activity in breast cancer. To enhance the immune system, take 1000 to 1500 milligrams daily. If you have breast cancer, take 8000 to 10,000 milligrams daily.

Shiitake (*Lentinus edodes*) contains a substance called lentinan, which stimulates production of natural killer cells. The recommended intake is 2 to 4 ounces of shiitake mushrooms two or three times per week. In rare instances, shiitake may cause temporary diarrhea and abdominal bloating if taken at high dosages.

Proanthocyanidins

Two other names often associated with this category of antioxidants are Pycnogenol and grapeseed extract. Pycnogenol is the patented name for the proanthocyanidins derived from pine bark. Compared with other antioxidants, Pycnogenol is 20 times more powerful than vitamin C and 50 times more powerful than vitamin E when it comes to destroying free radicals.

Grapeseed extract reportedly inhibits the growth of human breast cancer cells while enhancing the activity of normal cells. Take grapeseed extract in the form of OPC, or oligomeric proanthocyanidin, 100 milligrams daily, while undergoing radiation.

Rosemary

At the University of Illinois in Urbana, scientists experimented with extracts of rosemary (*Rosemarinus officinalis*), namely carnosol and ursolic acid. The carnosol, but not the ursolic acid, appears to prevent the growth of breast tumors, at least in rats. The study's investigators thus believe this component of rosemary may be a chemopreventive agent for breast cancer.

To prepare rosemary infusion, pour 8 ounces of boiling water over 2 grams of chopped rosemary herb. Cover and allow to steep for 15 minutes. Drink 2 to 3 cups daily.

Vitamin C

This popular antioxidant fights free-radical damage from carcinogens and increases the levels of white blood cells and interferon, another anticancer agent. If you are undergoing chemotherapy, vitamin C can help neutralize the free radicals formed by the drugs. High doses are recommended, but the best dose for you will depend on your tolerance level. Begin with 500 milligrams daily and increase by 500 milligrams every day or two until you experience gas and diarrhea. Then reduce the dose by 500 milligrams. This is your "tolerance" dosage.

Vitamin C comes in two different salts, sodium-L- and sodium-D-ascorbate, and as ascorbic acid. The salts are more effective than the acid when taken to alleviate the damage caused by the chemotherapy drug 5-fluorouracil (5-FU). If you have high blood pressure, however, avoid the salts. Ask your doctor about taking vitamin C before and during 5-FU treatment. The destructive effects of doxorubicin (Adriamycin) can be reversed by taking either form of vitamin C to tolerance level.

Vitamin E

Vitamin E is an antioxidant that can prevent damage from free radicals, protect heart muscle, help prevent baldness (a common side effect of chemotherapy and radiation), and help maintain white blood cell levels. Look for a supplement that contains vitamin E in the form of d-alpha tocopherol. Following are the dosage guidelines:

- If you are receiving chemotherapy or radiation, take 800 to 1600 international units daily. Monitor your blood pressure regularly. If it becomes elevated, reduce or stop taking vitamin E.

- Mouth sores (mucositis) are a common side effect of chemotherapy. Break open a 400–international unit vitamin E capsule and apply the oil directly on the sores.

- If you are taking Adriamycin, adding vitamin E appears to enhance the ability of the drug to kill cancer cells. High doses of vitamin E (1600 milligrams per day) may also help prevent the hair loss associated with the use of Adriamycin.

Natural Remedies for Benign Breast Conditions

If you are experiencing breast pain or tenderness, a breast infection, or breast lumps or cysts, there are several herbal, nutritional, and homeopathic remedies that can offer relief. Inform your physician when using these natural remedies. If you choose a homeopathic treatment, consult a homeopath for assistance. If water retention or swelling is part of the problem, you can try one or more of the herbal diuretics mentioned below.

HERBAL DIURETICS

ALFALFA *(Medicago sativa):* This herb relieves bloating and water retention and is an excellent source of phytoestrogens. To make an infusion, steep 1 to 2 teaspoons of dried leaves in 8 ounces of boiling water for 10 minutes. Drink up to 3 cups per day. For the extract, take ¼ teaspoon two to three times daily in water. Alfalfa is also available in capsules. Avoid alfalfa if you are pregnant or have lupus or anemia.

BLACK COHOSH *(Cimicifuga racemosa):* Black cohosh stimulates both estrogen and progesterone production and reduces water retention. For a decoction, add ½ teaspoon of powdered root to 8 ounces of water and boil for 30 minutes. Drink up to 1 cup a day, 2 tablespoons at a time. It is also available as a tincture, extract, and in capsules. Do not use black cohosh if you have a heart condition.

DANDELION *(Taraxacum officinale):* The roots of this popular "weed" are used as a diuretic. To prepare a decoction, place 1 heaping teaspoon of finely cut root into 16 ounces of boiling water and simmer for 15 minutes. Drink 1 to 2 cups a day. Do not take dandelion if you are pregnant or nursing.

PARSLEY *(Petroselinum crispum):* Along with dandelion, parsley is one of the most commonly used natural diuretics. To prepare an infusion, steep 1 to 2 teaspoons of dried leaves in 1 cup of boiling water for 10 minutes. Drink up to 3 cups a day. Parsley has no known side effects.

Breast Cysts

In addition to the natural remedies suggested below, eliminate caffeine, because its use has been associated with breast lumps (see Chapter 9):

- BURDOCK   Burdock root improves lymphatic flow and reverses abnormal cellular changes. Use 30 drops of tincture three to eight times daily, or drink 1 or more cups of infusion daily.

- FATTY ACIDS   Take two 500-milligram capsules of evening primrose oil three times daily, or 1 to 2 tablespoons of flaxseed oil, black currant oil, or hemp oil three times daily for 6 weeks.

- HOMEOPATHIC REMEDIES   Consult a homeopathic for dosing of belladonna, bryonia, graphites, pulsatilla, and/or conium.

- KELP   Take 1 tablespoon of kelp daily. Kelp contains iodine, and iodine deficiency is a common cause of fibrocystic breast changes. Also try other sea vegetables, including dulse, kombu, and wakame.

- POKE ROOT   Apply a poultice of puréed poke root and olive oil to the breast.

- RED CLOVER   According to Susun Weed and Christiane Northrup, in *Breast Cancer? Breast Health!* consistent use of red clover infusion can soften breast lumps and reverse precancerous conditions. Drink up to a quart of infusion daily. To prepare it, pour 32 ounces of boiling water over 8 to 12 teaspoons of dried flowers. Cover and steep for 10 to 15 minutes.

- VITAMIN E   Vitamin E helps circulate hormones to the breast and softens breast lumps. Some women report that vitamin E eliminates their cysts. Take 400 to 800 international units daily.

- VITAMIN B_6 Take 150 milligrams of vitamin B_6 daily for 10 days to 2 weeks before your menstrual period begins.

Fluctuating Hormone Levels

- CHASTEBERRY   Take 10 drops of chaste tree (vitex agnus castus) tincture diluted in water each morning during the second half of your menstrual cycle. For maximum benefit, also take 500 milligrams of evening primrose oil three times daily and 50 milligrams of vitamin B$_6$ once daily.

- CABBAGE   Place raw cabbage leaves inside your bra to help regulate hormone fluctuations. This old wives' tale apparently works for many women.

- DONG QUAI   Take 1 to 2 capsules of dong quai *(Angelica sinensis)* one to three times daily with meals (capsules usually contain 520 milligrams of herb). For the tincture, take ¼ teaspoon in ½ cup of warm water one to three times daily.

Mastalgia (Breast Pain)

In addition to the suggestions below, massaging the breasts from the chest outward can help eliminate excess milk in women who are breast-feeding, which can contribute to breast pain. Choose a private, quiet place where you can lie down. Use olive oil to make the massage easier. Start at the base of the breast or the chest wall and move slowly toward the nipple. Only apply as much pressure as is comfortable. Massage several times daily.

- CHASTEBERRY   A 1998 study of 97 women with severe breast pain showed that women who took 30 drops of vitex agnus castus (chasteberry) twice daily during three menstrual cycles experienced much quicker pain relief than did women who took a placebo.

- FENUGREEK   Add 8 ounces of boiling water to 1 tablespoon of fenugreek seeds and drink up to 3 cups daily.

Mastitis

If you experience fever, get plenty of rest and drink lots of fluids to help flush the infection from your system. Also follow the recommendations for echinacea and vitamin C below:

- CABBAGE   Place raw cabbage leaves in your bra to relieve the inflammation associated with mastitis.
- CALENDULA   Apply calendula cream to the nipples after every feeding.
- ECHINACEA   To help eliminate an acute infection, take 1 drop of tincture for every 2 pounds of body weight on the following schedule: dose every 2 hours for 1 to 2 days, then every 3 hours for 1 to 2 days, then every 4 hours for 1 to 2 days, then three times for a day, then twice a day, then once a day for a week.
- HOMEOPATHY   Homeopathic remedies include belladonna, bryonia, and phytolacca. Consult a homeopath.
- HONEYSUCKLE   A Chinese remedy uses honeysuckle (*Lonicera japonica*) to fight mastitis bacteria. Prepare a standard infusion using the dried flowers and drink 1 to 4 cups daily.
- LEMON   To help prevent infection, rub your nipples with lemon juice.
- POTATO   To draw out the heat of inflammation, make a poultice of grated raw potato and place on the breast.
- VITAMIN C   Take 1000 milligrams with bioflavonoids three times daily.
- VITAMIN E   Take 800 international units daily.

Nipple Pain

- CALENDULA   After breast-feeding, use a cool infusion of calendula on the nipples. To prepare an infusion, boil 8 ounces of water and pour it over 1 to 2 grams of the herb. Cover and allow to steep for 10 minutes. Cool before applying to the nipples. Or you can make a calendula compress. Soak a towel in the hot infusion, wring it out, and apply the compress to the breast. Cover the towel with a dry towel. Repeat the process when the compress cools. Calendula is also available as an ointment or cream.

- FENUGREEK   For inflamed nipples, grind fenugreek seeds and apply a hot poultice to the nipples.

- HOMEOPATHY   Remedies for cracked, sore nipples include castor equi, silicea, and graphites. Consult a homeopath for remedy selection and dosing.

- ST. JOHN'S WORT   After breast-feeding, rub dry nipples with 1 drop of St. John's wort oil diluted with 2 or 3 drops of olive oil.

- VITAMIN E   Because vitamin E helps repair skin tissue, it is helpful for sore nipples. Take 400 international units daily. You can also break open the capsules and squeeze the vitamin E oil directly on the nipples if they are cracked and dry.

Step 2 of the program shows how you can experience some impressive results when you tap into the healing power of Nature. And precisely because Nature's force can be so potent, it is important that you consult with and inform your physician or your medical management team when you introduce complementary approaches to your treatment plan. Many physicians are not familiar with some of the complementary remedies available for breast health care, so it may be up to you to share information with them. Strive to work with health professionals who respect your decision to seek complementary care.

CHAPTER SIX

Step 3: Deciding if Hormones Are Right for You

Every day, millions of women in North America take hormones in the form of birth-control pills (the pill), fertility drugs, or hormone replacement therapy. All of these hormones can have a big effect on breast health, as well as overall health. The problem, however, is that researchers don't always agree on what those effects are and whether they are beneficial or detrimental to a woman's health. And in the case of hormone replacement therapy, natural remedies and lifestyle changes are often the safer and equally effective approach.

The decision of whether to take hormones is a difficult one. That's why Step 3 is an important part of your program for breast health. This chapter presents information about the pill, fertility drugs, and hormone replacement therapy and the pros and cons of each. You should work closely with your health care practitioner during your decision process.

Oral Contraceptives and Breast Health

The pill has gone through many variations since it was first introduced in the 1960s. It was originally hailed as a safe, effective breakthrough in birth control, even when many of its side effects were not completely known or understood. Women who started with the first-generation pill received high doses of mestranol, a weak synthetic estrogen, along with a synthetic progesterone, or progestin. In the late 1970s, the second-generation pill was developed. It delivered lower doses of ethinyl estradiol, a very potent synthetic estrogen (40 times more powerful than the most active natural estrogen, estradiol), along with progestin. Third-generation pills are now available, and the majority provide a very low dose of estrogen and progestin. Other available hormonal contraceptives include medroxyprogesterone (injectable Depo-Provera), levonorgestrel (implant Norplant), and minipills (progestin-only pills). Each of these options contains varying amounts of hormones.

Early Health Concerns

In 1960, the year the first oral contraceptives hit the market, 800,000 women in the United States rushed to use them. By the mid-1990s, 75% of American women had used oral contraceptives at some point in their lives. Many of these women—and you may be among them—began taking the pill in their teens or early 20s and continued to use it for many years, some until they were in their 50s. And although there have been warnings to not smoke while taking the pill because of increased risk of blood clots, most believed they were taking a safe drug.

But the pill has had critics over the years. When Barbara Seaman, who eventually founded the National Women's Health Network, investigated the pill and its makers and published her findings in the book *The Doctors' Case Against the Pill* in 1969, it sparked a federal investigation. Seaman found that risks associated with use of oral contraceptives were being suppressed or dismissed by manufacturers, the U.S. government, and doctors. Dr. Hugh Davis of Johns Hopkins University told the U.S. Senate panel that "Never in history have so many individuals taken such potent drugs with so little information available as to the actual and potential hazards. The synthetic chemicals in the Pill are quite unnatural. . . . In using these agents, we are in fact embarked on a massive endocrinologic experiment with millions of healthy women."

The Studies

Although the number of women using oral contraceptives continued to rise throughout the 1970s and most of the 1980s regardless of the warnings from opponents, research into the possible health hazards of the pill was undertaken in earnest. Most of the studies done on the pill have been performed on first-generation products, because only they have been available long enough for researchers to conduct meaningful, long-term testing. From the earliest studies, there have been clear indications of a risk for breast cancer among women who use oral contraceptives. For example:

- 1977: A *Cancer* study showed an increased risk of breast cancer after only 2 to 4 years of taking the pill. The risk was greater for women with a history of benign breast problems.

- 1981: A 4-fold increased risk of breast cancer was reported in women younger than 33 years who had used the pill for 8 years before their first pregnancy.

- 1982: Another study found that women between the ages of 35 and 54 who had taken the pill before their first term pregnancy had three times the risk of breast cancer. The longer they had used the pill, the greater was their risk.

- 1986: A Scandinavian study published in *Lancet* reported that women younger than 45 had double the risk of breast cancer if they had taken the pill for more than 8 years before having their first child.

But in 1990, researchers at the Harvard School of Public Health in Boston conducted a study that disputed much of what had been said in previous work. Overall, they observed "no increase in the risk of breast cancer for women who had ever used oral contraceptives, even after long duration of use." They did find, however, a significant trend for increased risk among a small subgroup of premenopausal women who had used oral contraceptives for a long time, especially those who had used them for at least 4 years.

More studies followed, and most of them showed a significant risk for breast cancer associated with use of the pill. For example:

- 1995: A National Cancer Institute study headed by Dr. Louise Brinton reported that birth-control pill use increased the risk of breast cancer in women younger than 35 by 70%. Among women who had started using the pill before age 18 and who used it for more than 10 years, the risk was three times greater than for women who had never taken the pill.

- 1996: The Collaborative Group on Hormonal Factors in Breast Cancer evaluated the evidence from around the world on breast cancer risk and use of hormonal contraceptives. Its analysis of 54 studies included information on 53,297 women with breast cancer and 100,239 without it. The group reported that "the main findings are that there is a small increase in the risk of having breast cancer diagnosed in current users of combined oral contraceptives [containing both estrogen and progestin] and in women who had stopped use in the past 10 years but that there is no evidence of an increase in the risk more than 10 years after stopping use." Despite the large number of studies and women evaluated, the researchers still believed there was "insufficient information to comment reliably about the effects of specific types of oestrogen or of progestogen."

- 1998: At the University of Southern California, Los Angeles, researchers reported a 60% higher risk of breast cancer among women who had used high-dose estrogen for more than 12 years compared with nonusers, and a modest increased risk among women younger than 35 years and those with children who had started using the pill at a young age.

Review of Generations 1 and 2

What do all of these studies mean? Experts still do not fully understand the impact of oral contraceptives on breast health. One problem is that the majority of studies have been conducted on women who used first-generation products, even though third-generation pills are now available. As Samuel Epstein, M.D., and David Steinman report in their book *The Breast Cancer Prevention Program*, "The new Pill [second-generation] simply has not been around long enough for scientists to adequately assess its long-term safety. Moreover, the formula for the new Pill demands the use of progestin and the synthetic ethinyl estradiol; this means that although the amount is lower, the stimulatory effect is very much higher." Another problem is that many women have switched several times from one type of pill to another, and some have gone from taking birth-control pills to hormone replacement treatment.

Following her 1995 study, Dr. Louise Brinton of the National Cancer Institute noted that while experts thought they would see a "high risk of breast cancer associated with the use of high-estrogen-dose pills," like those that were prescribed between 1960 and 1975, "we haven't really seen that. Now we are beginning to think that maybe it's not the dose of the estrogen or the dose of the progestin; maybe it has something to do with the balance of the hormones." Perhaps the third-generation pills will hold the answer.

Some Good News

Today's third-generation oral contraceptives come in several forms:

- *Monophasic:* containing 1 milligram of progestin and 35 micrograms of estrogen, which are released at a steady rate throughout the monthly cycle.

- *Multiphasic:* come in two forms, *biphasic* and *triphasic.* The triphasic are the most prescribed form. Both multiphasic forms try to copy the fluctuating hormonal patterns of the menstrual cycle by providing very low doses of estrogen and progestin throughout the cycle.

The very low doses in these third-generation oral contraceptives may contain the right balance. At the July 1998 annual conference of the American Society for Reproductive Medicine, it was announced that the current oral contraceptives taken by more than 95% of women who are taking birth-control pills contain less than 50 micrograms of estrogen. Experts proclaimed these pills to be "remarkably safe," and said they do not increase a woman's risk of developing breast cancer. If this is true, it is good news for women who start taking the pill now. But for women who took the first- and second-generation pills, often for many years, the risk of breast cancer appears to be higher.

Birth Control Pills: Are They for You?

In 1990, the Food and Drug Administration (FDA) announced that the pill (third generation) was safe for women older than 35 if they did not have any of the potential risk factors for complications (smoking, history of blood clots, diabetes, high blood pressure). This paved the way for more women to take the pill longer. Some women may have started with first-generation pills, switched to second-generation products, and now continue on the third. Some started the pill in their teens, stopped in their 20s, and then started again in their late 30s or early 40s. Tracking the risk of breast cancer in these women will not be easy.

Should you take the pill? That's a decision you should reach along with your health care provider. Here are some factors to consider:

- Except for sterilization, it remains the single most effective method of birth control.

- Oral contraceptives that contain both estrogen and progestin offer protection against endometrial and ovarian cancer, and the longer you take the combination pill, the more protection you get.

- Once you stop taking the pill, the benefits appear to continue for about 15 years.

- The pill helps reduce the frequency of benign lumps and cysts in the breasts.

- You are at risk for complications from the pill (including stroke, heart problems, and worsening of an existing condition) if you smoke, have a history of blood clots, or have diabetes, asthma, liver disease, unexplained vaginal bleeding, high blood pressure, or cancer of the breast, uterus, or ovaries.

- Prolonged use of the pill may cause gallstones or difficulty becoming pregnant after discontinuing use.

Several contraceptives contain progestins alone. These include levonorgestrel (Norplant), which is implanted under the skin and prevents pregnancy for up to 5 years; Depo-Provera, an injectable progestin that prevents pregnancy for 3 months; and the minipill. If you are considering one of these contraceptives, review the facts:

- Studies show that women taking progestin-only contraceptives have a 30% increased risk of breast cancer.

- Even though no long-term studies of Norplant have been conducted, the contraceptive remains on the market. The FDA has received more than 6000 complaints about the contraceptive, with women reporting double vision, severe migraines, vomiting, heart attacks, stroke, and respiratory failure from use of the product. Other side effects include development of ovarian cysts, hair loss, and acne.

- Studies conducted with Depo-Provera show an increased risk of breast cancer after only a few years of use. In the *Journal of the American Medical Association*, for example, researchers reported that "women who started using [Depo-Provera] appeared to have an increased risk of breast cancer within 5 years." Other side effects include breast tenderness, loss of bone density, heavy bleeding, and weight gain.

- The minipill, which is slightly less effective as a contraceptive than pills that contain estrogen, causes menstrual cycle changes and ovarian cyst formation. It is recommended for women who are breast-feeding, women older than 35, and those with high blood pressure.

Alternatives to the Pill

Although all other birth-control methods (except sterilization) are less effective than the pill, some women choose nonhormonal approaches for contraception. These include the intrauterine device (IUD), diaphragm, vaginal sponge (not available in the U.S.), cervical cap, condoms, and spermicidal gels and foams. The gels and foams are the most effective when used in combination with the other methods.

Hormone Replacement Therapy

An estimated 31.2 million women were undergoing menopause in the year 2000, and that number will grow each year as more and more baby boomers turn 50, at the rate of one every 7.5 seconds! This means a large number of women are facing the need to make a decision that will greatly affect their current and future health: Should you take hormone replacement therapy? What are the risks? Now even more women are asking questions about hormone replacement, because some physicians are prescribing it to those who have had breast cancer and who are experiencing menopausal symptoms. There are no definitive answers to these questions.

Many women report feeling pressured by society and by their physicians to take hormone replacement therapy. If you pay attention to the advertisements for menopause medications and hormone replacement therapy, the underlying message is that menopause and postmenopause are illnesses. In our pill-pushing society, illness is treated with drugs; therefore, women need to "fix" this natural transition into their nonreproductive years.

Of course, women should seek relief for menopausal symptoms and should not ignore the real health risks (osteoporosis and heart disease) associated with the postmenopausal years. But there are alternatives to conventional hormone replacement therapy, and women should know what their options are when it comes time to tackle this issue. Before you look at the options, it helps to understand a bit about hormone therapy.

What It Means to Replace Your Hormones

Hormone replacement therapy is available in two main forms: estrogen only (estrogen replacement therapy, or ERT) and a combination of estrogen and progesterone (HRT), usually in the form of synthetic progesterone, or progestin. Most women who take estrogen also take progesterone or progestin. ERT is typically prescribed for women who have had their uterus removed. For women who still have their uterus, the progesterone in HRT helps the uterus shed endometrial cells, which in turn helps prevent the risk of endometrial cancer. However, progestin has been shown to increase the risk of breast cancer, so its inclusion in HRT is controversial. Both estrogen and progesterone stimulate breast cells, and they make breast cancers grow in laboratory animals.

Each form of hormone replacement therapy has its advantages and disadvantages, depending on your personal medical history and lifestyle. Whether the disadvantages outweigh the advantages depends on your particular situation. Here is what the research shows.

Estrogen Replacement Therapy

Estrogen is a broad term used to describe several related sex hormones in women—estradiol, estrone, and estriol. Estradiol is the most powerful and active of the estrogens. Any one or more of these estrogens can appear in ERT, and each form in turn may be included in a natural (chemically identical to the estrogens produced in the body) or synthetic (conjugated horse estrogen [Premarin], which is unnatural to the body) formula. Estrogen replacement therapy is available in pill form, as a cream, and in a transdermal patch.

Many studies show that ERT is associated with a significant risk of breast cancer. In 1991, for example, researchers evaluated eight studies and based on their findings they concluded that up to 8% of all cases of breast cancer among postmenopausal women could be attributed to use of ERT. Overall, the eight studies showed an increased risk of 20 to 80%. Another review of 16 studies placed the increased risk at 30%, with a 10-fold higher risk among women with a family history of breast cancer. In 1995, the Harvard Nurses' Health Study reported a 30 to 70% increased risk, which was followed by findings published in the *New England Journal of Medicine* in 1997 of a 43% increased risk of death from breast cancer among women who use ERT for more than 10 years. This study was based on data from 60,000 postmenopausal women.

If you take estrogen and also drink alcohol, your risk increases even more. Four to six ounces of alcohol a day along with ERT increases the body's estrogen levels by 300%.

Progesterone/Progestin Plus Estrogen: Hormone Replacement Therapy

Most women who take estrogen also use progesterone. Natural progesterone is derived from wild yam and because it cannot be regulated, physicians don't often recommend it. Synthetic progesterone, called progestin, is the most commonly used form. Although most people use the terms *progesterone* and *progestin* interchangeably, they are not the same and can cause different reactions.

Progesterone can be taken orally, although it is not very well absorbed; in a cream, which can be effective if the cream contains more than 400 milligrams/ounce; and as a suppository, which can be messy. In December 1998, the FDA approved an oral micronized progesterone for postmenopausal women. This form is better absorbed than the regular oral form. Researchers with the Postmenopausal Estrogen/Progestin Intervention trial (January 1999) "recommended oral micronized progesterone as the first choice for opposing estrogen in nonhysterectomized postmenopausal women." Micronized progesterone is very effective in preventing osteoporosis, may build bone, and can eliminate hot flashes without the need for estrogen. The only side effect was drowsiness, unlike progestins, which cause headache, depression, irritability, bloating, breast tenderness, and abdominal cramping.

HRT and Breast Cancer

Progesterone can inhibit cell reproduction in the breast and uterus, which leads some experts to believe the addition of progesterone to ERT may counteract the cell growth caused by estrogen. This benefit has not been proven, and, in fact, some past and recent studies indicate that the addition of progesterone increases the risk of breast cancer. It has been shown that both estrogen and progesterone stimulate breast cells and cause breast cancer cells to grow in laboratory animals.

In 1989, for example, the first study to evaluate the effects of combining estrogen and progestin was done in Sweden at the University Hospital in Uppsala. Researchers followed 23,244 women who took hormones after menopause. Two-thirds of the women took estrogen only and one-third took a combination product. Among the women who took estrogen only and developed breast cancer, their cancer rate was twice that of women who did not take hormones. Among those with breast cancer who took the combination hormones, the rate of breast cancer was four times as high as the rate among women who did not take hormones. (*Note:* This study has been criticized for not using a hormone combination commonly used in the United States and other countries and for not having enough women in the combination therapy.)

In 1992, Graham A. Colditz, M.D., reported a 59% increase in breast cancer risk among women who had used a combination hormone replacement therapy for more than 5 years. This risk increased by an additional 35% among women who were 55 years and older. A 1995 study in the *New England Journal of Medicine* showed a 40 to 60% increase in cancer risk.

More recent research has raised concern again. In January 2000, in the *Journal of the American Medical Association*, researchers reported on the results of the Breast Cancer Detection Demonstration Project. This study found that the combination of estrogen and progestin therapy may increase the risk of breast cancer beyond that of estrogen treatment alone. Their findings are the result of 15 years of follow-up of 46,355 postmenopausal women. The investigators point out that they saw a significantly increased risk among leaner women but not among heavier women. They also emphasize that further studies are needed to determine the accuracy of their findings.

Immediately after publication of this study, the *Journal of the National Cancer Institute* published study results stating that 5 years of HRT increase the risk of breast cancer by 24%, which is four times the risk from ERT alone. This research was conducted in more than 3,500 women.

The Dangers of Testosterone

Some physicians add testosterone to women's HRT to help increase sex drive. Several potential problems are associated with testosterone. One is that there are few long-term studies of the effects of this male hormone on women. Another is that a woman's fat converts testosterone into estrogen, which raises estrogen levels and thus the risk of breast cancer. Although research on the effects of testosterone in women is scarce, a 1996 study showed an increased risk of breast cancer among women who took the male hormone.

BENEFITS AND DISADVANTAGES OF ESTROGEN AND PROGESTERONE

Estrogen: Benefits

- Improves hot flashes, and vaginal dryness and itching.
- Reduces risk of urinary tract infections.
- Reduces risk of heart disease and osteoporosis.
- Reduces risk of Alzheimer's disease and colon cancer.
- Prevents blood coagulation.
- Helps maintain skin elasticity and tone and muscle mass.

Disadvantages

- Increases risk of ovarian and uterine cancers. According to Richard Theriault, medical oncologist and professor of medicine at M.D. Anderson Cancer Center in Houston, long-term use of ERT increases the risk of uterine cancer 15-fold. A 1995 study revealed a 40 to 70% increased risk of ovarian cancer among women using ERT for 6 years or more.
- Increases risk of endometrial cancer in women who have a uterus.
- Increases risk of gallbladder disease.
- Increases incidence of headache among women who suffer from migraines.
- Causes breast tenderness, bloating, nausea, weight gain, and vaginal bleeding.
- Can cause existing uterine fibroid tumors to become painful and to bleed.
- Can cause depression.

Progestin: Benefits

- Reduces risk of uterine cancer.
- Helps protect bone mass, although to a lesser degree than estrogen.
- Helps reduce hot flashes.

Disadvantages

- Can cause anxiety, severe depression, restlessness, and even psychosis in some women.
- Can cause acne, facial hair, and decreased sex drive.
- Often causes fluid retention, weight gain, and bloating.
- A January 2000 study in *Lancet* revealed that HRT makes it hard to detect breast cancer on mammography in women ages 50 to 69. This occurs because HRT increases tissue density, which makes it difficult to see cancer on a mammogram.

Note: Both estrogen and progesterone stimulate breast cells and have been shown to make breast cancer cells grow in laboratory animals.

Should Breast Cancer Survivors Take HRT?

If estrogen is a primary factor in whether a woman will get breast cancer, why would she want to take estrogen after she has had breast cancer? This question is being asked more and more often, as some physicians recommend HRT, primarily to help prevent osteoporosis and heart disease, to women who have had breast cancer. These women must weigh which risk is greater for them, given their personal and family histories: getting heart disease or osteoporosis, or having a recurrence of breast cancer.

The idea that some breast cancer survivors should take HRT is relatively new, and therefore there are no long-term data on the consequences. Based on the fact that there is no definitive evidence that taking HRT will cause breast cancer to recur, some doctors prescribe it to breast cancer survivors. Women who may be at greatest risk and therefore should not take HRT are those who have a genetic risk for breast cancer and those who had cancer with estrogen-positive receptors (see Chapter 10).

Yet other physicians strongly oppose giving HRT to any breast cancer survivor. Many of these doctors recommend alternatives, such as those described below. Ultimately, however, the decision to use HRT should be made between a woman and her physician, based on her past and current health, family history, and lifestyle.

Is Hormone Replacement Therapy for You?

Women usually choose to take HRT to prevent osteoporosis or to reduce their risk of heart disease. Below are the major risk factors for osteoporosis and heart disease. Note how many of these risk factors apply to you. Women who consider taking hormones for relief from symptoms of perimenopause and menopause alone very often can get that relief using natural approaches.

Consider the "Alternatives to HRT" below. Hormone replacement therapy can be your last choice when you know your options. Discuss the risks and alternatives with a health care provider who understands these alternatives.

Risks for Heart Disease

Family history of coronary artery disease

Total cholesterol above 200 mg/dL

Elevated triglycerides (above 200 mg/dL)

Lifestyle factors: inactivity, smoking, alcohol use

High dietary fat intake (more than 30% of total calories)

Diabetes

High blood pressure

Overweight

Remember: To effectively protect against heart disease, HRT needs to be taken indefinitely. After 10 years of estrogen, your risk of breast cancer increases about 30%.

Risks for Osteoporosis

Caucasian

Tall and slender

Advanced age

Early menopause (before age 40)

Family history of osteoporosis

Anorexia nervosa or bulimia

Low calcium intake

Lifestyle factors: inactivity, smoking, excessive use of alcohol, caffeine

Abnormal absence of menstruation

Prolonged use of corticosteroids and anticonvulsants

Alternatives to HRT

Adopting healthy habits or enhancing those you already practice can help you avoid the need for hormone replacement therapy. The alternatives to HRT explained below can also be used in conjunction with HRT if you and your health care provider decide you need hormones, perhaps for only a short time, while you establish your lifestyle changes:

- Eat a healthy diet (see Chapter 4) that includes lots of dark leafy greens and fresh fruits.

- To relieve menopausal symptoms, increase your intake of soy products and foods containing phytoestrogens.

- Monitor your protein intake. Most people eat too much

protein, and protein robs calcium from your body, contributing to osteoporosis.

- Take a calcium-magnesium supplement. The ratio of calcium to magnesium should be 2:1; thus, take 1000 to 1500 milligrams of calcium and 500 to 750 milligrams of magnesium daily.

- Take vitamins C and E to protect against heart disease and relieve menopausal symptoms (see Chapter 5).

- Exercise. As little as 30 minutes of aerobic exercise three times a week protects the heart and relieves menopausal symptoms (see Chapter 7).

- Consider botanical progesterone treatments. Botanical progesterone, which is derived from wild yam, is used to eliminate menopausal symptoms and to treat osteoporosis. According to John R. Lee, M.D., use of progesterone cream results in "a progressive increase in bone mineral density and definite clinical improvement including fracture prevention." He has found that "osteoporosis reversal is a clinical reality using a natural form of progesterone derived from yams that is safe, uncomplicated and inexpensive." See "For Further Reading" in the Resources, especially John R. Lee, M.D.; Christiane Northrup, M.D.; and Raquel Martin.

- Consider herbal remedies. Black cohosh, dong quai, and chaste berry, which are high in plant estrogens and progesterones, help balance hormone levels and treat menopausal symptoms. See Chapter 5 for dosing instructions.

- Consult a homeopath (or other health care professional knowledgeable about homeopathy) about remedies to relieve menopausal symptoms. Some of the remedies that may be recommended include aurum metallicum (for depression and vaginal dryness), lycopodium (for depression, low sex drive, and bloating), pulsatilla (for hot flashes, mood swings, and low sex drive), and sepia (for depression, bloating, and vaginal bleeding).

⚬ Reduce stress. There is evidence of a link between stress and breast cancer, and it is well known that stress is a factor in symptoms associated with menopause, including depression, mood swings, and irritability. Practice the stress-reduction methods described in Chapter 7, or consult "For Further Reading" to explore some of your own.

⚬ Find a physician who uses natural hormones. Contact the American College for Advancement in Medicine (1-800-532-3688) or the American Association of Naturopathic Physicians (1-206-298-0126).

If you are at high risk of osteoporosis and decide you need hormones, you can greatly reduce your risk of breast cancer if you start ERT after age 65. A study in the *Journal of the American Medical Association* revealed that women who delayed estrogen therapy for at least 10 years after menopause got the bone-conserving benefits of ERT that were similar to those in women who had begun treatment in their late 40s or early 50s.

Fertility Drugs and Breast Health

Whether a woman should take fertility drugs is a very personal and emotional issue, which is not addressed here. However, your decision must also take into account the medical impact such drugs can have on your health. This section offers information to consider as you make your decision.

What Are Fertility Drugs?

Fertility drugs are hormones, or substances that directly affect the action of hormones, which are taken to increase the chance that viable fertilization will take place. Clomiphene, a widely used fertility drug, is not a hormone but works by blocking estrogen. A progesterone called Crinone is also sometimes prescribed. Two fairly recent additions to the fertility drug scene are Pergonal, which is a combination of two hormones, FSH (follicle-stimulating hormone) and LH (luteinizing hormone); and Metrodin, which is LH alone.

Fertility Drugs and Cancer

Fertility drugs have been used with frequency only in recent years. That said, and the fact that it usually takes breast cancer 10 years or more to reach a detectable stage, along with the fact that the women who took fertility drugs in the late 1970s and early 1980s would now just be reaching menopausal age, there is little relevant research on any possible link between fertility drugs and breast cancer. But the results of the few recent studies show no association between the two. However, experts at Duke University observed that women who take fertility drugs are nine times more likely to develop ovarian cancer. They believe this cancer develops because of "incessant ovulation" prompted by the drugs rather than due to a direct action of the drugs themselves.

Fertility Drugs and Side Effects

Fertility drugs do affect the breasts, as well as other sites of the body. Women taking clomiphene may experience breast tenderness, bloating, hot flashes, headache, nausea, ovarian cysts, and the possibility of multiple pregnancy. Multiple pregnancy is also a risk for users of Pergonal, who may develop enlarged ovaries and pelvic pain. Women who take Crinone complain of swollen, tender breasts.

Before you decide to take the pill, ERT, HRT, or fertility drugs, do your homework. If you took the pill many years ago and now want to take it again, or if you are nearing menopause and are considering ERT or HRT, investigate the risks and your options. Taking hormones is a serious matter, and each woman has her own unique circumstances that need to be considered. Surround yourself with information and professionals to help you make your choice. Know that you have options, and discuss them with knowledgeable professionals. Ultimately, the choice is yours.

CHAPTER SEVEN

Step 4: Caring for Your Mind/Body

You are much more than your body: you are also mind and spirit, a holistic unit whose parts need to work together for optimal health. That's why Step 4 addresses the mind/body connection, a critical part of any health plan. This chapter looks at three factors that help keep all the parts working together in harmony and shows you how to create that balance for yourself. First it discusses the relationship between exercise and breast health and offers tips on how to make exercise a part of your routine, even if you have had breast surgery.

Next it explains how you can use yoga, meditation, and guided imagery to reduce stress, which are often part of recovery and support programs aimed at breast cancer survivors. Finally, you will learn about natural ways to eliminate known and potential carcinogens and other toxins that can harm your body and your breasts. Suggested detoxification methods you can use at home or can access through professionals are explained.

Moving Toward Breast Health

You've heard lots of reasons why it's important to exercise, and here's another one. Researchers have found that active women (4 hours of exercise per week) have a reduced risk of breast cancer. And the reduction is significant: in some studies, it was as high as 60%. If you find it hard to believe that jogging or attending an aerobics class several times a week can contribute to your breast health, read on.

The Studies

That exercise is beneficial to breast health is not new news. In 1985, the *British Journal of Cancer* reported that young women athletes had a lower prevalence of breast cancer than did nonathletes. This study was followed by several more in athletic women, all with the same findings. Naturally, not every woman is an athlete, but that isn't necessary. In a 1989 study of 7400 postmenopausal women, researchers found a 70% greater risk of breast cancer among inactive versus active women.

One thousand women younger than 40 were the focus of a National Cancer Institute study. The researchers found that the women who consistently exercised about 4 hours per week reduced their risk of developing premenopausal breast cancer by more than 50%. They got this benefit even if they didn't start to exercise until they were in their teens. If 4 hours sounds like a lot, even 2 to 3 hours reduces risk, but not as much—about 30%. The authors of the study emphasized that "continued participation in a physical exercise regimen can markedly reduce the risk of breast cancer in premenopausal women" and stressed "the importance of beginning an exercise regimen early in life and maintaining it through adulthood."

Why Exercise Reduces Risk

Experts believe several factors contribute to the reduction in breast cancer risk among women who exercise. If a young girl is active, exercise can delay menarche, which reduces the number of years estrogen will surge through her system. Studies show that a girl needs at least 17% body fat for menarche to begin. Women who exercise and keep their body fat levels lower than 22% typically have lower estrogen levels and are less likely to ovulate, even when they continue to menstruate regularly.

Active women tend to experience early menopause, which also reduces the estrogen levels. Exercise increases the level of estrogen-binding proteins, which attract the hormone away from the estrogen receptors in the breast cells. Activity also limits the conversion of testosterone to estrogen. Studies also find that athletic women tend to eat diets that are low in fat and have little or no meat. These eating habits are associated with lower levels of estrogen.

Finally, exercise helps control weight. The more fat you have, the higher your estrogen level; thus, maintaining optimal weight is key in the prevention of breast cancer. It's interesting that higher levels of body fat are associated with a greater risk of breast cancer among postmenopausal but not among pre-menopausal women (see Chapter 10). However, being over-weight at any age is unhealthy, and it is rare for women who are overweight before menopause to lose their excess weight after menopause. In fact, throughout adulthood, women typi-cally gain 5 to 10 pounds per decade, which means many women are overweight when they reach postmenopause. Thus, exercising to help maintain a healthy weight is your best bet.

Get Up off the Couch

It's up to you to get off the couch; no one can do it for you. It also is not the purpose of this book to give you exercise rou-tines. If you need suggestions, consult some of the many books on the market about aerobic exercise (see "For Further Read-ing" in the Resources for recommendations). After that, the guidelines are simple:

- Choose exercise(s) that you enjoy. If you hate to run, don't do it just because your friends like it. Bike, walk, swim, dance, do aerobics, ski, play tennis.

- Vary your exercise. Walk two days, bike one, play tennis another. Avoid boredom.

- Exercise with a friend.

- Consult your physician if you are over 35 and/or haven't exercised in a long time.

- If it's not fun, make it fun. Turn on some music, get a radio, listen to books on tape. If you need motivation, join an aerobics class or a walking club at an area indoor mall.

Exercise After Breast Surgery

After breast surgery, women face a time of emotional, spiritual, and physical recovery. Depending on the extent and type of surgery, regained mobility in the arms and the amount of pain will vary. Physicians typically prescribe specific exercises after breast cancer surgery to help women regain mobility and strength in their arms. Among women who have their lymph nodes removed, some experience lymphedema (see below), which is a buildup of lymph fluids in the arm and chest area that causes pain and limits movement and range of the arm and sometimes the hand. Along with massage and manual lymph drainage, which are discussed below, exercises facilitate recovery. Exercise also helps soften scar tissue so that movement will be easier. If you have undergone breast surgery, your physician will provide you with an exercise program.

Below are four simple arm exercises that are typical of those recommended after breast surgery. Do each of the exercises five times, three times a day. Ask your doctor which movements are best for your condition and when you can start. Most physicians encourage women to begin mild exercises within 48 hours of surgery:

- Stand with your feet comfortably apart or sit straight up in a chair. Extend your arms in front of you with palms facing and elbows straight. Stretch your arms above your head and link your fingers. Slowly bend your elbows and clasp your fingers at the back of your neck. Push your elbows back as far as possible, then pull your elbows toward each other. Repeat.

- Sit or stand with your hands folded behind your back and slide them up as far as possible.
- Place your hands on your shoulders and move your elbows up sideways as far as possible, then down.
- With your hands on your shoulders, make circular movements with your elbows. Make as large a circle as possible, then change direction.

The following exercises can be started after your stitches have been removed:

- Stand close to a wall, facing it, and place your fingertips on it. Creep up the wall, like a spider, using your fingers, as high as you can go. Try to increase the height each time you do this until your arms are straight.
- Stand next to a chair with one foot (the side opposite to the surgical side) in front of the other. Hold onto the back of a chair while you lean forward and swing the arm on the side of the operation side to side, then back and forth, as far as is comfortable. Increase the amount of swing until the arm reaches shoulder height. Keep your elbows straight. You can add a small hand weight as you progress.
- Begin in the same starting position as the exercise above. When you lean forward this time, swing your arm on the side of the operation in circles, first clockwise and then counterclockwise.

Reducing Stress

Experts have established that improper management of stress—and not necessarily the amount of stress you experience—plays a significant role in overall health. Breast health is no exception. For well-being, you need to manage the stress in your life. Below are three effective and easy ways to reduce stress—meditation, visualization and guided imagery, and yoga—as well as information about support groups. It is recommended that you incorporate one of these, or another of your choice, into your lifestyle. To help you do that, several sample sessions are included.

Stress and Breast Cancer

Researchers in the evolving field of psychoneuroimmunology, which explores the intimate connection between the mind/body and health, have discovered a link between stress and cancer. Much of the relationship hinges on how you perceive stress and then react to it, because your perception influences how your body will respond.

During times of stress, the body kicks into "fight-or-flight" mode, marked by a quickened heartbeat, rapid breathing, and the release of stress hormones such as adrenaline, norepinephrine, and cortisol. This response was meant to be short-lived. But in today's world the fight-or-flight mode often goes on endlessly or is repeated again and again, weakening the immune system. Staying in high-stress mode with elevated levels of stress hormones can compromise the immune system and has been linked to many diseases, including breast cancer.

Some interesting studies have been done to determine the effect of stress reduction on women who have breast cancer. For example, psychiatrist Dr. David Spiegel reported on a 10-year study in which he tracked the progress of women with metastasized breast cancer. He found that the women who had taken part in therapeutic support groups lived nearly twice as long as women who had not attended therapy sessions. Similar results have been found in many other studies of the effects of stress reduction on cancer in general.

Scientists are not certain exactly how or why reduced stress has a positive effect on health in general and cancer in partic-

ular. However, the ever-evolving field of psychoneuroimmunology continues to make discoveries that will hopefully
solve this mystery.

A Breathing Exercise for You

Regardless of the stress management approach you choose,
proper breathing plays an integral role. The breathing exercise
explained here is just one of several approaches you can use.
(For other techniques, see "For Further Reading.") Use this
breathing exercise as a prelude to the exercises in this chapter.
Also practice it several times a day whenever you feel the need
to relieve tension:

1. Place the tip of your tongue against the ridge behind and
   above your upper front teeth. Allow it to remain there
   throughout the entire exercise.
2. Exhale completely through your mouth, making a
   "whoosh" sound as the air leaves you.
3. Keep your mouth closed as you inhale deeply and quietly
   through your nose to a count of 4.
4. Hold your breath for a count of 7.
5. Exhale through your mouth to a count of 8, making a
   "whoosh" sound.
6. Repeat steps 3, 4, and 5 for a total of four breaths.

During the first month you practice this breathing exercise,
limit the number of breaths to four at one time, but you can
practice several times a day. After a month, increase to eight
breaths each time if you wish.

Meditation

With the help of medical professionals such as Bernie Siegel,
M.D., who has done extensive research on the benefits of meditation in medicine; Herbert Benson, M.D., who introduced
the concept of the relaxation response; and Jon Kabat-Zinn,
Ph.D., director of the Stress Reduction Clinic at the Univer-

sity of Massachusetts Medical Center, meditation has moved out of the alternative arena into the mainstream. Meditation allows you to focus your mind in a state of relaxed and heightened consciousness and perception for the purpose of achieving a restful trance that unburdens and strengthens the mind. Meditation has been likened to watching a parade: You allow images and thoughts to pass through your consciousness, but you do not act on them or think about them. This approach is unlike guided imagery (discussed below), in which you use the images to reach a specified state of awareness.

How Meditation Works

Meditation lowers the level of stress hormones in the blood, lowers blood pressure and blood sugar levels, and reduces heart and breathing rates. These changes occur as the body enters a state of relaxation. For many people, meditation also has a spiritual component, which is a source of healing for them. Scientists have proven that this state of calm exists by elevating the alpha brain waves (the waves associated with deep relaxation and creativity) of people who meditate.

Types of Meditation

The two basic types of meditation are mindfulness (or insight meditation) and concentrative, and each one has several variations. Once you understand the basics of each type, you can decide which one best suits your needs, or use them both.

MINDFULNESS MEDITATION   The expression "being in the moment," expresses the essence of mindfulness meditation. Mindfulness is about being fully aware in the present moment and accepting each moment as it is. Think of the parade analogy: You allow yourself to be aware of the feelings and thoughts that pass through your mind, but you do not allow yourself to think about them or to join in.

One of the masters of mindfulness mediation, Jon Kabat-Zinn, Ph.D., explains that it helps people see a situation as it is and to accept it. This can be helpful for women who have breast cancer. Dr. Kabat-Zinn believes that when people accept their situation, they are better able to respond effectively to it.

CONCENTRATIVE MEDITATION   In the 1970s, Drs. Herbert Benson and R. Keith Wallace studied concentrative meditation and successfully used it to reduce heart rate and breathing rate. Concentrative meditation involves focusing on a repetitive image, sound, or action, which in turn helps quiet the mind and heighten awareness. One of the most familiar repetitive sounds used in concentrative meditation is the humming sound "ohmmmmmmmm," commonly referred to as a mantra. Focusing on the breath or a flickering candle are other common practices.

How You Can Use Meditation

Meditation can be used to relieve stress; to alleviate pain associated with premenstrual syndrome (PMS) and menopause, such as breast tenderness and breast pain; and as a complementary remedy for cancer pain. To get the most benefit, meditation should be practiced daily. Some cancer support groups make meditation part of their regular program. In addition to helping relieve physical discomfort and pain, meditation can help you get a new perspective on your life and provide a sense of spiritual well-being.

Once you become adept at meditation, you can do it anytime, anywhere. Beginners often like to assume the standard meditative pose (see below), but it is not necessary. Use any position that is most comfortable for you.

MEDITATION POSE

- Sit on the floor with your legs straight out in front of you, forming a V shape.
- Bend your right leg and bring it toward you. Place your right foot on the floor close to your groin.

- Bend your left leg and place your left foot on the floor close to your right leg.
- Rest your hands on your knees: arms outstretched and palms up.
- Keep your back straight.

Meditation can be learned from an instructor, from tapes, or from books. Many people use meditation tapes because they are convenient. Below are two brief meditation exercises: one for breast pain and tenderness and one for stress relief. You can tape these scripts; you also can record meditation scripts from other books, purchase prerecorded meditations, or borrow them from your public library (see Resources).

Mindfulness Meditation for Breast Pain

- Get into a comfortable position, lying down if possible. Use pillows, blankets, or whatever you need.

- Slowly stretch from your head to your toes so that you feel completely present in your body. As you stretch, take a body inventory. Start with your toes and acknowledge each body part as you mentally move up your body. If you reach a part that is uncomfortable, tender, or painful, simply acknowledge the discomfort without making any judgment about it. Continue your inventory until you reach the top of your head.

- Close your eyes if they aren't closed already and take a deep, slow breath. Exhale slowly and completely, making a whooshing sound if you like.

- As you take your next deep breath, focus on a spot just below your navel. For a few minutes, send each breath to that spot. Be aware of each breath as it reaches the spot and as it leaves.

- Now allow yourself to shift your attention away from that spot and to become fully aware of your body. Focus on the spot in your breast that bothers you. If more than one spot is a problem, concentrate on only one at a time. Deal with each site completely before you focus on another one.

- Take a deep breath and send it to the problem area. As you inhale, be aware of any sensations in or around the spot— pain, burning, aching, tenderness. Simply be aware of the sensations; do not judge them or think about them. They are not good or bad—they simply are.

- As you exhale, notice if the sensations change. Acknowledge any sensations and let them be. Allow your breath to sweep over the problem spot as it leaves your body. Continue to breathe in and out, slowly and gently, acknowledging any sensations that come to you. Continue to breathe into that site until you feel some relief.

- If you have another problem area of your breast that needs attention, focus on sending your breath to it. Repeat the process above.

- After you have focused on all of the areas that needed attention, take several deep breaths, release them slowly, and open your eyes as you return to full consciousness.

It may take several sessions before you get significant stress relief or pain reduction. Like most things, meditation takes practice, and the more you do it the better your results will be.

Concentrative Meditation for Stress Reduction

1. Choose a meditation pose that is most comfortable for you.

2. Close your eyes and allow your body to relax. If you are lying down, allow your weight to sink into the floor. If you are sitting, lift your chest and let your chin fall lightly toward your throat. Place your hands on your knees, palms up. If you choose, touch the tips of your thumb and index finger of each hand.

3. Inhale deeply and slowly through your nose. Hold the breath for a few seconds and then exhale slowly. Repeat

this cycle for about 2 minutes. At the end of each exhale, squeeze your buttocks and hold the squeeze for a few seconds. Concentrate only on your breath and the squeeze.

4. After you repeat this cycle for 2 minutes, switch your focus to any place in your body where you are feeling tense or your muscles are tight. Meditate on that spot and focus on sending your breath deeply into it. See that spot clearly in your mind. Continue to meditate on that spot and breathe deeply for about 2 minutes. With every exhale, send the tension out of your body.

5. Choose another uncomfortable site and focus on it. Repeat the cycle in step 4.

Visualization and Guided Imagery

You can use the power of the images in your mind to relieve breast pain and tenderness, to eliminate stress, to facilitate healing after breast surgery, and to help prevent breast cancer recurrence. Visualization and guided imagery are powerful mind/body techniques that are quickly becoming accepted among mainstream medical professionals. Although some people are skeptical about using guided imagery for healing, it is completely safe and may provide many benefits, as long as it is used to complement, and not replace, conventional therapy.

To better appreciate guided imagery, it helps to understand visualization, which is the preface to guided imagery. Visualization is a way to use one or more mental visual images (sometimes called the "mind's eye") to achieve a specific goal; for example, to relieve tension and stress, to heal physical or emotional disease, or to alleviate pain or discomfort. In guided imagery you bring together those images and incorporate your other senses as well, to create scenarios in your mind—like a mind-movie—that support your goal.

In *Staying Well with Guided Imagery: How to Harness the Power of Your Imagination for Health and Healing*, author Belleruth Naparstek explains that guided imagery is "the deliberate production of healing sensory images." For guided imagery to be effective, you need to place yourself in an altered state of consciousness using self-hypnosis. If you have never tried self-hypnosis, don't worry. Most people find it easy to do after a few sessions. Attaining an altered state of consciousness is a key factor for why guided imagery is effective.

Using Guided Imagery

The images you use during your guided imagery sessions are unique because they are the products of your imagination, experiences, and dreams. There are no right or wrong visions. If you are new to guided imagery, you can get tapes to help you. You can also read scripts of guided imagery sessions in books and use them as they are or modify them to your needs. An example of such a script is below. It is a suggested approach to dealing with breast pain.

If you would like to do guided imagery to deal with breast cancer, refer to "For Further Reading" and "Products for Breast Health" (at the back of this book) for sources of scripts. One approach to deal with disease involves cellular imaging, in which you focus on your body's activities at the cellular level. To be effective, this technique requires that you have a basic understanding of breast cancer and how cells function. Advocates of this type of guided imagery believe that the mind can influence cell function. For more information, see books by Bernie Siegel, M.D.; Martin Rossman, M.D.; and Michael Samuels and N. Samuels in "For Further Reading."

Why Does Guided Imagery Work?

One reason guided imagery is effective is because the mind has a powerful influence over the human body. You can use your mind to trick your body into responding in certain ways based on the images your mind conjures up. For example, the body can't distinguish between a real lemon and an imaginary one. If you don't believe it, try this: Close your eyes and visualize a lemon. In your mind, cut the lemon in half and place one-half of the fruit into your mouth. Picture yourself sucking on the lemon. Can you imagine the sourness? Did your lips pucker involuntarily? You have just used guided imagery, and your body reacted to an imaginary lemon.

Another reason guided imagery works is because being in an altered state of consciousness and highly focused calm alertness gives you an increased ability to heal and learn. When you feel helpless and out of control, it has a negative effect on your self-esteem, your energy level, your immune system, and other aspects of your life. Guided imagery allows you to regain some control over your pain and your life.

The Studies

Only a few studies have explored how guided imagery helps relieve pain and fight disease. Pioneers in the field include O. Carl and Stephanie Simonton, who taught people with cancer how to use guided imagery to manage their disease. Some patients claim their tumors have shrunk or disappeared completely after using guided imagery over time, yet there are no scientifically controlled studies to back their claims.

Most patients who use guided imagery report great relief from anxiety and pain, and a feeling of control over their disease. Scientists hope to have documented proof of these benefits some day. Perhaps Patricia Newton, M.D., of Portland, Oregon, will be one such researcher. She received a grant from the National Institutes of Health (NIH) Office of Alternative Medicine to study whether mental imagery and hypnosis can enhance the immune system response of women with breast cancer.

Several studies have suggested this trend. At Stanford University, psychiatrist David Spiegel evaluated the impact of guided imagery and hypnosis on 86 women with breast cancer. He divided the group into two subgroups. Both groups received the same medical treatment but only one group was taught guided imagery and self-hypnosis. After 1 year, the women in the guided imagery group reported having much less pain and fewer mood swings, and a greater sense of control. This group also lived an average of twice as long as the other group.

In Britain, women who practiced guided imagery while they received chemotherapy for breast cancer enjoyed a better quality of life than women who did not use imagery. At the University of Akron, Ohio, researchers found that "guided imagery is an effective intervention for enhancing comfort of women undergoing radiation therapy for early stage breast cancer."

Guided Imagery for Breast Pain

Here is a guided imagery script to relieve stress and tension. Feel free to modify it:

Choose a comfortable, quiet location where you can be alone for 10 to 20 minutes. The position you choose is not important as long as you are comfortable. Close your eyes and keep them closed throughout the session.

To begin, breathe in slowly to a count of 6 and then release the breath slowly to a count of 6. Repeat several times.

Tighten the muscles in your toes to a slow count of 4, and then release. Continue to breathe slowly and deeply throughout the session.

Each time you breathe in, imagine you are taking in the present. When you breathe out, you are releasing tension, stress, pain, worries, and fears. Notice any sensations you may feel in your hands, feet, arms, neck, shoulders, and legs as you breathe in and out.

Tighten the muscles in your calves to a slow count of 4 and then release.

Continue to move up your body, tightening your muscles to a count of 4 and then releasing them. Do this for your thighs, buttocks, abdomen, forearms, hands, shoulders, face, and neck. Continue to release tension and other unpleasant feelings as you breathe out.

Once you finish this part of the exercise, picture a place where you feel at peace. Choose any place, real or imaginary: perhaps a place you've been or one you'd like to visit; a place you've read about or one you'd create if you could.

Allow yourself to enter that place and be a part of it. Inhale every smell and identify it. Tune in to every sound you hear. Savor the taste of any food or beverage that may be sharing the space with you. Reach out and feel the textures, forms, warmth, coolness, and essence of everything in your special place.

Notice every color and hue around you. See how the light plays on the contours and casts shadows. Feel the air on your skin or the sun on your face or whatever surrounds you in this special place. Surrender to the richness of all that is around you.

Take a deep breath and allow the serenity of your special place to reach into every cell in your body. Allow that peace to wash over you and through you with warmth and softness.

With every deep breath, fill yourself with calmness and tranquillity. With every exhale, release tension and discomfort and allow it to dissolve or drift away in a breeze.

Continue to breathe in deeply and exhale easily, releasing tension and negative feelings as you exhale. Know that with each deep breath you inhale healing energy and that with each exhale you release darkness.

Knowing that you can return to your special place whenever you need to and that it will always embrace you with healing energy, you bid it farewell as you continue to breathe easily and slowly. Gradually return to your starting point, slowly opening your eyes when you are ready, knowing that now you are more energized and in control of all that you are.

Support Groups

Stress reduction is important for everyone, but especially for those who are undergoing treatment for breast cancer. Breast cancer support groups can help women cope with the emotional, spiritual, and physical stress associated with the disease.

Several studies of the impact of breast cancer support groups reveal the benefits women get from these gatherings. In one 1997 study, women reported that they gained an "enhanced sense of control, sharing of information and experiences, and acquaintance with positive role models." A *Psychooncology* study found that participants in breast cancer support groups reported them to be "extremely helpful for navigating the short and long-term impact of breast cancer." For information about groups in your area, contact your local American Cancer Society or refer to the listings in the Resources.

Yoga

Yoga (which means "yoking") is a system of breathing, movements, and postures that has been practiced for more than 5000 years. The practice was developed to harmonize and integrate the body, mind, and spirit in a balanced state of higher consciousness. Although there are many variations of yoga, the most common ones share the elements of stretching (*asanas*), breathing, meditation, and spiritual enlightenment. Specific postures and positions are used as therapy to promote healing. Because yoga works simultaneously on the body, mind, and spirit, it is especially suited for this purpose.

Many breast cancer support and therapy groups incorporate yoga into their programs. The programs teach specific postures and movements that help women who have had breast cancer surgery. If you are interested in trying yoga, contact a case worker at the hospital where your surgery was performed, the American Cancer Society, or a local cancer support group for information on sessions in your area. Consult your physician before starting yoga.

Inner Cleansing: Detoxification

No matter how hard you try to avoid them, toxins are everywhere, and your body takes them in. As you will discover in Chapter 9, these toxins play a significant role in causing breast cancer and in affecting your overall health. Once carcinogens enter your body, they attach themselves to fatty cells, tissues, and organs, where they can cause damage. Breast tissue, with its wealth of fat cells and estrogen receptors, is a prime breeding site for uncontrolled growth of cells, or cancer.

Detoxification is the process of removing toxins from the body. The body's ability to cleanse itself is a major indicator of how healthy it is. Because poisons constantly enter the body, you need to remove them continuously. Detoxification can reduce the risk of cancer, boost energy, enhance the immune system, slow the aging process, eliminate aches and pains, relieve allergy symptoms, and improve other areas of your health.

Some ways to eliminate toxins from your body include juice and herbal fasts, enemas, saunas, colonics, and massage. The Gerson Diet Program (Chapter 4), for example, uses both juice cleansing and enemas for detoxification. These two techniques address the two main organs involved in the detoxification process: the liver and the intestines.

The Role of the Liver and the Intestines

The liver is the largest organ in the body. At any one time, about 25% of all the blood in the body is circulating through the liver—nearly 2 quarts every minute. This occurs so that the liver can break down and detoxify substances from the blood that can be toxic to the body, such as pesticides, medications, food additives, saturated fats, alcohol, and other poisons. Once it processes these substances, it eliminates them or finds a way for the body to use them. The intestinal tract is one of the main vehicles for elimination of these toxins; the kidneys are another.

If the liver cannot properly break down toxins and wastes because of disease or nutritional deficiencies, or because it is overburdened, they can get into the bloodstream and slowly poison the body. Many toxins are fat soluble, which means once they reach the fatty cell membranes, they attach themselves and can cause cancer. Because the breasts are composed primarily of fat cells, they are prime sites for the buildup of toxins.

Daily Detoxification

Because your body is constantly exposed to harmful substances, detoxification needs to be an ongoing practice. One way to assist the body in eliminating toxins is to eat a diet that focuses on fresh fruits and vegetables, whole grains, legumes, and nuts and seeds, organic when possible. Drinking at least eight glasses of filtered water every day is another good practice.

You can add specific supplements and herbs to your diet to help rid your body of toxins. The following herbs will help you do just that. Those that help clear the lymphatic system are especially useful for breast health. When you are not fasting, use one or more of the herbs daily, either as a supplement (extract, capsule, or tincture) or as an infusion or decoction (see pages 95–96 for an explanation of terms). These herbs can be used during a juice and herb fast, when you can enjoy several cups of your favorite infusion or decoction daily.

Herbs for Detoxification

- BURDOCK ROOT *(Arctium lappa):* This burr-bearing herb is both a diuretic and a choleretic (stimulates removal of bile). It helps cleanse the blood and liver and assists in the elimination of toxins through the kidneys. To make a decoction, add 1 teaspoon of root to 24 ounces of boiling water. Cover and steep for 30 minutes. Drink 1 to 2 cups daily at room temperature.

- DANDELION ROOT *(Taraxacum officinale):* This "weed" is an excellent diuretic. It stimulates the elimination of toxins from every cell in the body and promotes secretions from the liver. To prepare a decoction, boil 2 to 3 teaspoons of powdered root in 1 cup of water for 15 minutes. Let it cool.

For an infusion, place ½ teaspoon of dried leaves in 1 cup of boiling water and let it steep for 15 minutes. Drink up to 3 cups daily of either remedy.

- LEMON BALM *(Melissa officinalis):* Lemon balm helps cleanse the lymphatic system. Prepare an infusion by pouring 8 ounces of boiling water over 1 to 3 teaspoons of balm leaves. Cover and steep for 10 minutes. Drink 2 to 3 cups per day.

- MILK THISTLE *(Silybum marianum):* This herb protects the liver against damaging effects of chemicals, medications, radiation, pollutants, and alcohol, and promotes drainage of the liver. The most effective form is the capsule; follow package directions. It is also available as a tincture: take 10 to 40 drops in water up to three times a day.

- UVA URSI *(Arctostaphylos uva-ursi):* This herb cleanses the lymphatic system and the spleen. To prepare an infusion, boil 16 ounces of water and let it cool slightly. Pour the water over 1 ounce of herb and let it steep for 15 minutes. Drink up to 3 cups daily at room temperature. To use the tincture, take 10 to 30 drops in water up to three times a day.

- YELLOW DOCK *(Rumex crispus):* This herb cleanses the liver, blood, and lymphatic system, and also helps remove toxins through the kidneys. Loose stools are a rare side effect. To prepare an infusion, pour 16 ounces of boiling water over 1 to 2 teaspoons of dried herb. Cover and steep for 10 minutes. Drink 3 cups daily. For the tincture, take 3 to 4 milliliters in water three times daily.

Supplements That Support Detoxification

The following supplements support detoxification. Include them as part of your daily supplement plan. Some health care professionals recommend abstaining from supplements during a juice and herb fast:

- Lipotropic agents, which include choline, betaine, methionine, folic acid, and vitamins B_6 and B_{12}, stimulate the flow of bile and fat through the liver. You can buy a lipotropic formula or take the supplement SAM-e (S-adenosyl-L-methionine) along with folic acid and vitamins B_6 and B_{12}. A lipotropic agent should provide 1000 milligrams of choline and 1000 milligrams of either methionine or cysteine daily. If you take SAM-e, take 600 to 800 milligrams.

- Vitamin B complex, 100 milligrams daily.

- Spirulina, wheatgrass, or barley grass, 1 tablespoon daily, to help cleanse and rebuild tissue.

- Coenzyme Q10, 100 milligrams daily.

Detoxification Through Fasting

Fasting has been practiced for millennia for both cleansing and therapeutic purposes. Michael Murray, N.D., author of *The Encyclopedia of Natural Medicine*, recommends going on a 3-day juice fast four times a year. Some nutritional experts recommend taking specific herbs during a juice fast, like those mentioned above, either as teas or supplements. In any case, filtered water is an essential part of any detoxification plan.

Sensible fasting allows the body to heal, to produce new healthy cells, and to resist toxins and infections. Most people think that fasting means totally abstaining from food and liquids, yet complete abstinence causes the rapid release of the toxins stored in the fat cells and organs, which can cause problems during the fast and afterward. Thus, most medical experts recommend juice and herb fasts for healing purposes, especially if it is your first or second fast.

Sample Detoxification Fast

During a juice and water fast, it is important to support your body's detoxification efforts. Guidelines for a recommended approach to a 3-day fresh juice fast are below. Consult your health care provider before starting the fast:

- On the day before you start your fast, your last meal should be composed of only fresh fruits and vegetables.

- Purchase a juicer. Purchase one that can withstand the rigors of vegetables such as carrots and beets. The best models leave the fiber in the juice. Ask friends for referrals.

- Drink three or four 8- to 12-ounce glasses of freshly prepared fruit and/or vegetable juice per day of the fast (recipes below). Organic produce is preferred.

- Avoid coffee, bottled, canned, or frozen juice, or soft drinks during your fast. Herbal teas can be added, but do not use sugar or sweeteners.

- Drink at least four 8-ounce glasses of filtered water per day of the fast.

- Some experts recommend taking a high-potency multi-vitamin-mineral supplement once daily and 1000 milligrams of vitamin C three times daily during a juice fast. Others disagree, saying that supplements interfere with detoxification and that the nutrients in the juices are more than adequate. Consult a trusted nutritionist on this question.

- Take 1 to 2 teaspoons of powdered psyllium seed husks, guar gum, oat bran, or another natural water-soluble fiber a half hour before each meal with plenty of water. Begin with less fiber and work up gradually to this amount.

- Take silymarin, 70 to 210 milligrams three times daily.

- Mild exercise, such as a short walk or light stretching, is acceptable, but do not exert yourself. This is a healing, restful time, and exertion hinders the detoxification process.

- Because your body temperature, blood pressure, pulse, and respiration rate will probably decline, it is important to stay warm.

- Rest is important. Take naps.

- On the first day after your fast is over, eat fruit for breakfast and a vegetable salad for lunch.

- On day 2 postfast, repeat breakfast and lunch from day 1 and add vegetable soup for dinner.
- On day 3 postfast, have larger portions of fruit and vegetables, add nuts, baked potato, and squash.
- On the fourth day, return to your normal diet.

BASIC JUICES FOR FASTING

Vegetable Broth

In a large pot, place 1½ quarts of water and chop or grate the following vegetables: 2 large red potatoes (organic, leave skins on), 3 stalks celery, 3 medium beets, 4 carrots, one-half head green or red cabbage, 2 turnips, 1 red onion, 1 cup turnip or beet tops. Season with your favorite herbs and simmer, covered, for 45 minutes. Cool slightly, then pulse in a blender. Drink warm.

Green Fruity Juice

Take 16 ounces of any combination of the following fresh juices: orange, grapefruit, pineapple, lemon, tangerine. Add to it 1 cup of any of the following (or ½ cup of two different additions): celery, radish tops, burdock, parsley, chard, dandelion, sprouts, carrot tops, wheatgrass, raspberry leaves. Place in a juicer and pulse until well blended. Drink cool.

Detoxification Baths

Toxins can be eliminated through the skin, and a detoxification bath is an easy and relaxing way to do this at home. If you are routinely exposed to high levels of pollutants, take weekly detox baths for a month or two, then one every 2 to 4 weeks.

A detox bath includes the use of bath additives (see below), which help draw the toxins from the body. If you take frequent detox baths, switch among the additives you use because they can lose their effectiveness if the same ones are used all the time. This is not true of Epsom salts, which can be used solely if you desire. Here are the guidelines for a detox bath:

- Before you enter the detox bath, use a loofah sponge or a rough washcloth and mild soap to scrub the oils and dead skin from your body.

- Drink at least 8 ounces of water.

- Fill the tub with hot water to a level that allows you to immerse your entire body except your head. Make the water as hot as you can tolerate without burning yourself.

- For your first detox bath, stay in the water for 5 minutes only. You may feel some effects from the bath, such as dizziness or light-headedness, immediately or hours later. Have someone available to help you get out of the tub safely should you need assistance.

- For subsequent detox baths, stay in the water for 5 minutes longer each time until you reach 30 minutes. Take two or three baths each week until your health improves.

- Immediately after getting out of the water, shower to remove the toxins from your skin. Your body will reabsorb any toxins you fail to remove.

BATH ADDITIVES   Choose from the following bath additives. If you are taking detox baths several times a week, rotate the additives. If you use Epsom salts for each bath, there is no need to switch:

- Apple cider vinegar: Pour ¼ cup vinegar into your bath water the first time. Increase the amount by ¼ cup each time until you reach 1 cup. Vinegar increases blood flow to the skin.

- Burdock root: Place one handful of burdock root into a large pot with 2 quarts of water. Simmer for 30 minutes, strain, and add the infusion to a tub of hot water. Burdock root helps eliminate uric acid from the body.

- Epsom salts: Each time you use Epsom salts, increase the amount you put into the tub of hot water by ¼ cup. Start with ¼ cup and increase until you reach 4 cups. Epsom salts increases perspiration and changes the pH balance of the skin.

- Herbs: Prepare an infusion of any one of the following herbs and add 1 cup to the tub water to promote detoxification: boneset, chamomile, blue vervain, catnip, peppermint, horsetail.

- Salt and soda: If you have been exposed to radiation, this is an effective detox bath. Add ½ pound of baking soda alone or along with ½ pound of sea salt to each bath.

Manual Lymphatic Drainage

A therapeutic technique called manual lymphatic drainage (MLD) is a massage method that stimulates the flow of lymphatic fluid through the lymph system. It was developed by physical therapists Emil and Estrid Vodder in the 1930s. Lymph fluid moves and eliminates accumulated waste and toxic substances from the body and supplies the tissues with white blood cells. When the flow of lymph is obstructed because of injury, illness, or because some of the nodes have been removed, swelling can result. This occurs because, unlike the blood, which is pumped through the body by contractions of the heart, lymph fluids rely on muscle contractions, the pulse of arteries, and external body movements to flow through the body. Manual lymphatic drainage promotes the flow of lymph fluid. Long-term treatment can soften scar tissue and restore tissue elasticity.

Removal of some lymph nodes is common in breast cancer surgery, and in most cases does not cause serious problems. But in about 5% of cases their removal can cause a chronic, painful condition known as lymphedema. Symptoms include swelling of the fingers and arm, and depending on the extent of the swelling, it can severely limit movement. Manual lymphatic drainage can be used to eliminate lymphedema, but more importantly it can be used to prevent it.

Manual lymphatic drainage should be done by a therapist who is specially trained in the technique. Look for a practitioner who knows how to work with women who have undergone breast cancer surgery. See Resources for finding a professional MLD therapist.

Saunas

A sauna is an effective way to release toxins from fat cells. Saunas can be either wet or dry, and the dry version is better for detoxification because it increases sweating and therefore accelerates the detoxification process. An effective sauna detoxification program includes 20 minutes of exercise, followed by up to 30 minutes in a dry sauna and a cleansing shower to wash away the toxins. Both during and after the sauna, drink plenty of water to help flush the toxins from your kidneys. If possible, have a massage after your shower.

If you are pregnant or think you could be, do not use a sauna. If you begin to feel light-headed while in the sauna and you have been drinking enough water, leave the sauna. Drink extra water and rest until the feeling passes, but do not return to the sauna that day.

Step 4 has introduced you to several ways to obtain and maintain a balance between mind and body. Some of the ideas may have been completely foreign to you. Perhaps you've considered meditation, and now you have a reason to try it. Maybe you're thinking twice about the pollution you're exposed to every day and are intrigued by the idea of a juice fast. Hopefully your interest has been piqued enough for you to take action. You owe it to yourself to strive for health.

CHAPTER EIGHT

Step 5: Breast Screening and Preventive Maintenance

You've seen the public service advertisements. You've heard advice from various cancer groups, and you know they're right. Routine examining of your breasts should be part of your overall breast health program. But are you doing it?

Step 5 of your breast health program includes breast self-examination (BSE), yearly breast examination by a qualified health care professional, and mammography or another screening option, when applicable. The importance of these steps cannot be overemphasized. When and how these measures should be taken, at what age you should start, how long you should continue them, and how regularly you should do them are discussed in this chapter. Included are the debates and controversies about the necessity, safety, and accuracy of mammography.

You may be surprised to learn that there are alternatives to mammography. Most women believe that besides physical examinations, mammography is the only way to screen for breast cancer. The truth is, there are several screening options, and this chapter introduces them to you.

A point that must be emphasized is that although regularly doing any of these screening procedures can mean the difference between life and death, they *do not* prevent breast cancer. Any information that claims these methods prevent breast cancer is false and misleading. These procedures are screening techniques only, designed to detect breast abnormalities so that you can take early and immediate action. In that sense, they help prevent more serious disease.

This chapter also takes a look at the brassiere: its evolution, and whether it is healthy or necessary to wear one. Do bras promote breast health? What are the facts behind stories that bras can cause breast cancer? You'll learn some things about bras that will help you make the best selection.

Breast Cancer Detection Guidelines

On March 23, 1997, the American Cancer Society Board of Directors revised the society's guidelines for detecting breast cancer in women without symptoms of the disease. The modified guidelines are as follows:

- Women 20 years and older should perform BSE monthly.
- Women 20 to 39 should have a breast physical examination every 3 years by a health care professional.
- Women 40 years and older should have a physical examination of the breast every year by a health care professional and a yearly mammogram.

Not everyone agrees with the American Cancer Society's guidelines. Some experts argue that teens should do BSE to get them into a good habit early. Others say that because breast cancer is rare in younger women, starting BSE at age 25 is sufficient. But the most controversy is around the issue of the mammography guidelines. Who the dissenters are and how they feel about mammography are discussed below under "Mammography," followed by information about alternative screening procedures. Once you have the information, it's up to you and your health care professional to arrive at the best screening approach for you.

Breast Self-examination

In this age of high-tech computers and medical technology, one of the best screening techniques for detection of breast cancer doesn't involve computer chips or even electricity. Breast self-examination is a simple, noninvasive, completely private screening approach that many experts believe is highly effective in detecting breast cancers. The reason experts can only "believe" it is effective is because there are no large, well-controlled studies that have proven this to be the case. The studies that have been done suggest a drop in breast cancer death rates of 25 to 35%. And most health experts agree that BSE is one of the best ways a woman can take control of her breast health.

The World Health Organization is hoping to have a definitive answer from the study it is sponsoring. More than 193,000 Russian women ages 40 to 64 are involved in a 15-year study to determine whether BSE significantly reduces the death rate from breast cancer. Unfortunately, results of the study will not be available until around 2010.

Why BSE Is Important

No one knows your breasts better than you do. But you can't know them unless you do routine examinations. When you examine your breasts periodically, you get to know them well and will be best able to detect any changes. The National Cancer Institute states that women who do careful, routine BSE are able to detect lumps as small as one-quarter to one-half of an inch. Any suspicious lump should be checked by your physician. The majority of these lumps are benign fluid-filled cysts or fibrocystic lumps (see Chapter 11). If, however, your doctor determines that the lump is cancerous, early detection is your best ally. Breast cancer that is diagnosed in its early stages can usually be handled with a lumpectomy, which conserves the breast (see Chapter 10).

Why Women Resist BSE

The idea that a woman can detect her own breast cancer is both frightening and empowering, but unfortunately many women perceive it to be much more of the former. Indeed, fear is the primary reason why women do not do routine BSE. Many say they are afraid they will find a lump or other abnormality. Certainly women don't want to find breast cancer, but if it is there, early detection could very well save their lives. Besides, more than 80% of lumps are benign: a nuisance, perhaps even painful, but not cancerous.

Some women say they don't do BSE because they don't know how or because they're afraid they will miss finding a lump, and these excuses are related to fear. Any woman who wants to learn how to do BSE can simply ask her physician or nurse practitioner to teach her; or she can contact any one of the cancer organizations, or pick up a book at the library. Fear of not doing it right or missing a lump can be alleviated by getting instruction on BSE from your physician, nurse practitioner, or a breast cancer educator. There are also products on the market that help women learn how to do BSE so that they will feel confident they are doing a thorough job (see "Getting to Know Your Breasts" below).

"Isn't it my doctor's job to check my breasts?" say some women. Yes, but he or she probably only gets the opportunity to do so once a year if you're good about scheduling regular yearly gynecologic exams. If you get a professional breast examination in January and you do BSE and find something questionable in March, isn't it better to have it checked out right away instead of waiting until the following January for your next appointment? Breast health is a partnership: the doctor does his or her part, but you need to do yours as well.

"I don't have time to do BSE" is another common excuse, but it only takes about 10 to 15 minutes per month. It's time well spent to help ensure your good health. Some women feel uncomfortable or self-conscious touching their breasts, perhaps because they were taught that it is wrong to look at or touch their body. If you feel this way, approach BSE slowly. Try doing it while wearing a thin blouse, or create a relaxing mood with music in a space where you feel safe.

Getting to Know Your Breasts

If you are in your reproductive years, the best time to do your monthly BSE is during the first week after your period. During this time, your estrogen and progesterone levels aren't high and your milk glands and ducts are not swollen. Once your estrogen and progesterone levels begin to rise during the second week after your period, swelling of the glands and ducts will make your breasts feel lumpy and tender and thus much harder to examine properly. If you are postmenopausal, your breasts are most likely less lumpy and are not affected by fluctuating hormone levels. In this case, choose the same, convenient time each month to do your exam, say, the first day of each month.

The first few times you do BSE, you will familiarize yourself with how your breasts feel and establish a point of reference, so you will be able to tell whether anything unusual appears later. Many women are surprised to discover that their breasts feel like cottage cheese—lumpy all over, or in certain spots. This is normal, which is the reason why it is best to examine your breasts during the first week after your period, when lumpiness is minimal. You may also notice that your breasts are not exactly the same size and that one breast is higher on the chest than the other. These are perfectly normal and common characteristics.

One fear is not being able to determine the difference between normal lumpiness and a detectable growth. Women used to be told, "You'll know the difference when you feel it," but today there is an easier way. Many doctors, clinics, and hospitals have silicone breast models called *MammaCare*, which allow women to learn how to feel the difference between normal lumpiness and growths. A health care professional can help you practice on the models until you feel confident. (See Resources for information on MammaCare.) There are also special pads (e.g., SensorPad) you can place over your breast that can help you examine your breasts more accurately.

Doing BSE

Breast self-examination doesn't take any special instruments. If you can schedule a breast examination with a professional who can guide you the first time you do BSE, that's good. If not, don't wait until you get an appointment. Follow the guidelines below, and if you have any questions about the procedure, call your doctor, nurse practitioner, or breast cancer educator.

What Am I Looking For?

During both visual and tactile (touching) inspection, there are several things you will look for. It's important, however, that you first know what is normal for your breasts so that you have something with which to compare. For example, some women have one or both nipples inverted, and this is normal for them. But if your nipples have always been everted (stick out) and you notice during BSE that one of your nipples is inverted and it remains that way, that is a change you need to report to your physician. During BSE you look for changes in your breasts from what is normal for you.

During your visual inspection, look for dimpling of the breast, bulges in the contour of the breast, puffiness or swelling, reddened areas, prominent blood vessels, rash or sores on the nipples, or fluid emitted from the nipple when it is squeezed gently. Any of these changes may be caused by simple fluctuations in fluid in the breast, weight gain or loss, or a harmless cyst. To be safe, report changes to your health care professional.

How to Do BSE

Visual Examination

1. Stand or sit in front of a mirror in which you can see your entire torso. Keep your arms relaxed at your sides. Note the shape, color, texture, symmetry, and other characteristics of your breasts. Pay attention to your nipples and areolas for skin tone, rashes, puckering, or other traits.

2. Turn slowly. As you bring one breast forward, note any changes in the contour of the breast. Then turn the other way and view the other breast.

3. To look for dimpling or swellings, raise your arms above your head, or clasp your hands behind your head. This allows the muscles in your chest to tighten and elevates your breasts. Turn slowly, first to one side, then the other, to view your breasts.

4. Place your hands on your hips and bend forward at the hips so that your breasts hang straight down. (If you are sitting, you will need to stand for this part.) Note if your breasts hang symmetrically and if there is any change in size.

5. If your breasts are large, lift each breast with the opposite hand to inspect under the breasts.

Tactile Examination

1. Lie on a bed or other flat, comfortable surface. You may do BSE while lying on your back or on your side, whichever is more comfortable.

2. If your breasts tend to bulge to the sides when you lie flat, place a pillow under your shoulder as you examine each side.

3. To examine your right breast, place your right arm behind your head.

4. There are three main patterns you can use to palpate (feel) your breasts—vertical strip, circular, and wedge. The vertical strip is the technique found to be the most effective and is the one taught in many hospitals and clinics. It is sometimes described as mowing the lawn, using an up and down pattern and overlapping the rows as you go. It is the method explained below. (See the figure for all three methods.)

5. Using your left hand, press the pads of the three middle fingers against the skin immediately under your collarbone and near your shoulder.

6. Using a firm, small rotary motion, press on the surface of the breast, then with a bit more pressure, and then more again, all the while remaining in the same location.

7. Continue to feel along an imaginary bra line down the outside of your breast. At the bottom of your bra line, you may feel a ridge of hard tissue. This is normal.

8. When you reach the bottom of your bra line, slide your fingers toward your nipple about one-half inch and continue your examination by working back up toward your collarbone.

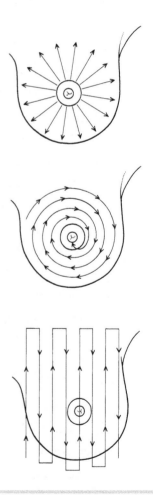

The BSE Technique for Breast Palpation

9. Continue until you reach your breastbone in the center of your chest. Repeat the examination on the left breast. Remember to place your left arm behind your head.

10. Gently squeeze the nipple of each breast to check for discharge.

11. When you are done with the vertical strip examination, stand or sit in front of a mirror with your arms relaxed at your sides. Visually examine your breasts for anything abnormal.

According to the U.S. Department of Health and Human Services, 50% of lumps are found in the upper, outer portion of the breast. This is where the breast tissue is most dense. Eighteen percent appear in the nipple area, 15% in the upper, inner portion of the breast, 11% in the lower, outer portion, and 6% in the lower, inner area. Don't let this information stop you from examining both breasts in their entirety, however.

BSE in Special Circumstances

Breast self-examinations should be done by all women. Situations such as pregnancy and breast-feeding, breast surgery, and breast implantation should not exclude women from doing BSE. Here are a few tips for these special circumstances:

- Pregnancy: Expect your breasts to be lumpy, but you should be able to feel any abnormality. If you do notice a lump, contact your physician immediately. Breast cancer discovered during pregnancy can be aggressive. To avoid exposing the fetus to radiation, ultrasound can be used to view the lump. If the growth cannot be identified, mammography may be necessary.

- Breast-feeding: The best time to do BSE is when the breasts are empty of milk.

- Breast surgery: Before undergoing surgery, do BSE and make a mental note of how the breasts feel. This will give you a basis for comparison when you feel the scar tissue from the operation.

- Breast implants: Insertion of breast implants will leave scar tissue around the incision and perhaps around the implant as well. Familiarize yourself with your breasts before implant surgery so that you can identify the scar tissue later. Some experts recommend undergoing an MRI every few years to check for leakage from the implants.

What to Do If You Find a Lump

If you find a lump that doesn't feel right to you, contact your physician for a more thorough examination. On average, a lump that is one-half inch in diameter (1 centimeter) probably has been growing for 10 years to reach that size. This is important information, because if the growth does turn out to be cancerous, you need to know that you don't have to make an instant decision about treatment. You should not wait months, but take a week or two to get a second opinion, consult with more than one breast specialist, research your case, and then make an informed decision. A few weeks' delay is not likely to change the outcome, and you will feel confident that you have acted wisely.

Breast Examinations by Your Doctor

The breast examinations done by your doctor, physician's assistant, nurse, or nurse practitioner are in addition to those you do yourself and are just as important. The recommendations of the American Cancer Society are for women who have no symptoms of breast cancer or other breast problems. Any woman who has symptoms should seek immediate medical attention.

When the examiner is well trained and takes his or her time with the clinical breast examination, the detection rate can be up to 87%. This is also a good time to ask any questions you have about BSE and to pay attention to the technique used by the practitioner.

Mammography

It seems that every few months another study about the pros or cons of mammography is reported in the media. Not every medical organization or physician agrees with the American Cancer Society's guidelines for mammography. In fact, most of the rest of the world does not recommend breast cancer screening using mammography before age 50. Among the organizations that adhere to the 50-plus guideline are the American College of Physicians, European Group for Breast Cancer Screening, the Canadian Task Force on Periodic Health Examinations, the International Union Against Breast Cancer, and the U.S. Preventive Service Task Force. The National Cancer Institute is in between: it recommends mammograms every 1 to 2 years for women older than 40 and suggests that women older than 40 who have a family history of breast cancer discuss the possible need for more frequent screenings with their physician.

What Should I Do About Mammography?

The debate about mammograms—when, how often, and even if you should get them at all—leaves many women confused about what to do. These are questions women need to answer with the help of a trusted health care provider. It also helps to know the information on which experts base their opinions.

Numerous studies back up the beliefs of the above organizations. A study published in *Current Clinical Trials* showed that screening women younger than 50 is of little value. Another study found that mammography was unable to detect more than half the breast cancer treated in premenopausal women. Similarly, the Breast Cancer Action organization conducted a survey in which it found that only 37% of women with breast cancer had their disease detected using mammography.

In August 1999, a *Cancer* report from an international team of investigators stated that women younger than 50 should be screened for breast cancer every 12 to 18 months. Their rationale: Breast cancer progresses more quickly in younger than in older women, so screening should be more frequent. The experts studied more than 77,000 women. They reported that yearly screening for women ages 40 to 54 would reduce mortality from breast cancer by 32%.

Pros and Cons of Mammography

Mammography has its fans and dissenters, and there are reasons for both. First, the good news. Statistics show that women 50 years and older who undergo mammography screening are 30% less likely to die of breast cancer. This significant fact is one reason why mammography is considered to be the gold standard in breast cancer screening by many experts. About 40% of all breast cancers are found through mammography, and another 35% are discovered during a combination of physical examination and mammography. Masses as small as one-fifth of an inch (0.5 cm) can be detected through mammography.

Now the less positive news. Even if you have the best radiologic technician do the screening using the best equipment, an estimated 10 to 15% of cancers, or more, are missed. Even when a mass is discovered, a mammogram cannot identify whether it is benign or malignant. Mammography also is not effective in detecting abnormalities in dense breast tissue, which are normal in women younger than 50.

Alternative Screening Methods

Digital Mammography

An alternative to regular mammography is digital mammography. Although it still emits radiation, the images are clearer, and unlike traditional mammograms, the images can be enhanced. This ability helps reduce the need for repeat images. Digital mammography images are stored electronically and can be easily transmitted anywhere in the world for consultation. The Food and Drug Administration (FDA) approved digital mammography for general use on January 31, 2000, although it will be some time before the procedure is widely available.

Magnetic Resonance Imaging

Another screening method that does not involve radiation is magnetic resonance imaging, or MRI. An MRI machine contains a magnet that activates the hydrogen molecules in the breast. Radio waves are transmitted to the magnet, which transmits information about abnormal tissue to a computer. Sometimes an injection of dye is used to distinguish a tumor. MRIs are especially useful for women who have silicone breast implants, because the high density of the silicone blocks 22 to 83% of breast tissue from a mammogram. MRIs are also recommended for women who have saline breast implants and for women who are considering breast-conserving surgery for breast cancer.

Positron Emission Tomography

Positron emission tomography, or PET, involves injection of a radioisotope, a dye that releases a nuclear substance called a positron. The isotopes are taken in by cells in the breast and lymph nodes and form "hot spots," areas where cancer cells are growing. The radiologist takes a series of images (tomograms), which are then put together to form a complete picture of the breast. PET provides clear pictures of very dense breasts, which is a plus for some women, but it also exposes the breasts to radiation.

Scintimammography

Scintimammography was approved by the FDA in May 1997 with the hope that it would help reduce the number of biopsies performed each year. Scintimammography involves the use of a radioactive tracer that is injected into the arm vein. This tracer contains technetium 99m, a synthetic substance that emits gamma rays; and a large molecule called methoxy isobutyl isonitrile. About 5 minutes after receiving the tracer, the woman lies on a special table that allows her breasts to hang freely as a camera takes several views.

On the plus side, research indicates that scintimammography is more than 90% accurate in detecting breast cancer, which is better than mammography. However, scintimammography exposes the breasts to the same amount of radiation used during mammography, and it is not sensitive to masses less than 1 centimeter in diameter. Some experts are concerned that the radioactive tracer may damage the ovaries, although there is no proof at this time.

Thermography

A diagnostic thermograph of the breast is a picture of the heat emitted from the breast. It is a painless, noninvasive procedure that does not involve radiation or injections. Also known as infrared imaging, this method can detect a precancerous condition in the breast up to 10 years before a cancerous tumor can be detected using any other approach. It is very sensitive (82%) in the detection of stage 0 and 1 cancers.

Thermography is not perfect. It has an overall 12% false positive rate (meaning that 12% of women without a cancerous tumor will get a positive test result), and it is not able to identify the exact location of a tumor. If, however, you want to avoid radiation and prefer an early warning of possible breast problems, thermography may be your choice.

The Bra: Use It or Lose It?

The idea of not wearing a bra was popular as a social statement in the 1960s, but could there be a medical reason as well? You may decide to ban your bra after reading the following section.

Confining and supporting the female breast is a relatively new concept. Before the 1400s, women's breasts were free, but with the advent of the Renaissance came changes in clothing styles and attitudes. First came the corset, which went through various styles and forms. Each modification seemed to push the breasts up and out more and more until it seemed nothing could contain them, including the low-cut bodices that were all the fashion at the time.

When the French Revolution arrived, the corset and low bodices went out of fashion until the Napoleonic age, when they made a comeback. More wars and social upheavals came and went, and along with them eventually went the corset.

The first bra was invented in the late 1800s by Mary Tucek, who got her "breast supporter" patented in 1893. It was very similar to the modern bra and had separate pockets for each breast. In 1914, a device that flattened the breasts rather than supported them was patented by Mary Phelps Jacobs. This design, though less like the modern version, was called a brassiere.

The influence of Hollywood and movies on female sexuality was overwhelming during the 1940s and 1950s. Marilyn Monroe and other well-endowed female icons were live advertisements for the new definition of sexy. Then during the 1960s, some women fought back against the bra as a symbol of male oppression. The braless look was followed and accompanied by a slowly growing acceptance of breast implants and breast cosmetic surgery.

Although bras are still "in," are they necessary, or even healthy? Some researchers say no to both counts.

Bras and Breast Cancer: Is There a Connection?

In 1995, a book entitled *Dressed to Kill* posed an intriguing idea: that wearing a bra may cause breast cancer. The authors, Sydney Ross Singer and Soma Grismaijer, based their claim on the Bra and Breast Cancer Study (BBCS), as well as existing medical data.

The link between the bra and breast cancer, according to the researchers, involves the effect of the bras on the lymph system. Because of the way bras are designed and the way the weight of the breasts is distributed, the lymphatic system cannot properly eliminate the toxins that build up or repair tissue damage. The shoulder straps, for example, may hinder drainage to the lymphatics that run from the armpit to the top of the breast. Bras that have underwires may hinder drainage to the lymph nodes in the breastbone.

The authors of *Dressed to Kill* propose that "constriction of the lymphatics may cause toxins to become concentrated within the breast tissue." Even though most women remove their bras at night, they are worn for about 16 hours a day. Thus, say the researchers, the chronic constriction of the breast tissue eventually may cause some breast cells to become malignant.

Many doctors are skeptical of these findings, including Gordon F. Schwartz, M.D., of Jefferson Medical College in Philadelphia, who says, "Even when a bra fits snugly, it doesn't interfere with the lymphatic drainage of the breast." Singer and Grismaijer reportedly are conducting a new study, this time including medical doctors in the research.

How to Choose a Fitting Bra

Most women in North America wear a bra, and as long as they do, it makes sense to ensure it is the most comfortable, functional, and safe bra possible. Here are some guidelines on how to get a well-fitting bra. (Take the following measurements while you are wearing a bra.)

- Measure your chest above your breasts and just below your armpits. This is your bra size.
- Measure your chest around your nipple area. This determines your cup size.

Compare the two measurements. If they are the same, you need an AA cup. If your cup size measurement is 1 inch bigger than your bra size, you need an A cup; 2 inches bigger, a B cup; 3 inches bigger, a C cup; 4 inches bigger, a D cup.

Once you choose the correct size bra, put it on and look in a mirror. You have a correct fit if:

- With your arms at your sides, your breasts lie halfway between your shoulder and elbow.
- There's a close fit at the breastbone.
- There's enough space to insert a finger under each cup.
- The back strap aligns with the base of the cups.
- The cups do not wrinkle.
- The straps do not cause indentations in your shoulders.

The best indication that your bra is the right size is how it feels after wearing it for a few hours. Different bra styles may fit differently, even when they are the same size. If your breasts change size significantly during your menstrual cycle, you may need different bras for those times, or you may purchase your bras to fit that time of the month when your breasts are most full.

Responsible breast care includes policing your breasts for potential problems. Consider your routine BSE and professional breast screenings to be part of your Five-Step Program for Breast Health. A little routine attention can be your best insurance against possible problems in the future.

※

CHAPTER NINE

How Food, Alcohol, Caffeine, and Environmental Factors Affect Breast Health

A common misconception about breast cancer is that heredity plays a major role in whether women will develop the disease. Yet only about 5% of women with breast cancer have a family history of the disease. The vast majority of cases—75% or more—are attributed to diet, lifestyle, and environmental factors. Exactly what percentage each of these factors plays in breast cancer is not known for certain, but researchers have determined their significance for cancer in general. According to the *Harvard Report on Cancer Prevention*, 77% of all cancers are related to lifestyle, including diet, obesity, stress, amount of exercise, tobacco and alcohol use, occupational risks, and food contamination. Genetic and related risk factors are believed to be responsible for 14%. That leaves 9% to be attributed to environmental causes, such as air, water, and soil pollution, household and industrial chemicals, radiation, and perhaps even electromagnetic fields.

In this chapter you'll learn about the impact that diet, lifestyle, and environment may have on your breast health.

That's a lot to cover in one chapter, so we've narrowed it down to potential and proven carcinogens such as caffeine, alcohol, sugar, food additives, fats, pesticides and other environmental pollutants, radiation, electromagnetic fields, and the risks that specific occupations may carry for breast cancer.

One thing becomes clear: regardless of which possible carcinogen is discussed, scientists do not agree on the role it plays in breast cancer. Controversy and debate abound, which is good, because it fuels more research that will hopefully answer more questions about breast health.

Impact of Food- and Drug-Related Substances on Breast Health

How many cups of coffee or cans of cola do you drink each day? Do you have more than one alcoholic drink a day? Do you smoke? Is your idea of breakfast a donut and coffee? Does the majority of the food you eat come from a box, can, jar, or the fast food drive-up window?

No one is saying you will get breast cancer if you infrequently do any of these things. Rather, if they are habits, experts believe you are at increased risk for breast cancer.

But the news is not all bad. In fact, the goal of this chapter is not to simply tell you what to avoid but to explain how and why certain everyday items can be harmful to breast health, to discuss the extent to which they are believed to be harmful, and then to suggest healthy alternatives.

Caffeine

Caffeine is safe. Caffeine is bad. Caffeine consumption leads to breast lumps, cysts, tenderness, and pain. Caffeine is nothing to worry about. You've probably heard these comments and more about caffeine and breast health. If you're confused, you're not alone. Researchers themselves are uncertain about the exact connection between caffeine and breast changes. But research and anecdotal reports combined point to a definite relationship. Most of the research has focused on coffee, but if you drink caffeinated tea or colas, the risk is the same.

Caffeine and Breast Lumps

An association between caffeine and breast health was first recognized in 1979. Dr. John Minton of Ohio State University Hospital reported that breast lumps, tenderness, and pain had disappeared in 65% of his patients not long after they had eliminated all caffeine products from their diet. That number rose to 83% two years later when he did a follow-up study.

PRODUCTS CONTAINING CAFFEINE

Beverages   Coffee, tea, cola, Dr. Pepper, Mello Yello, Mountain Dew, Mr. Pibb, Tab

Foods   Cocoa, chocolate

OTC Drugs   Anacin, NoDoz, Excedrin

Prescription Drugs   Cafergot, Darvon, Fiorinal, Synalgos-DC, Wigraine

Since the 1980s, little research has focused on the impact of caffeine on breast health. Yet many physicians advise their patients to avoid foods and beverages that contain caffeine, because their patients tell them that when they do, they get relief from breast pain, tenderness, and lumps. These and other similar breast changes are discussed in Chapter 11.

Caffeine and Breast Cancer

No definitive link between caffeine consumption and breast cancer has been found, although caffeine does stimulate breast cancer growth in some mice species. Caffeine belongs to a class of chemicals called methylxanthines, which have been linked to cancer in laboratory animals. But in human studies of more than 45,000 women, no connection between caffeine intake and breast cancer has been found.

The Bottom Line

Caffeine apparently has a detrimental effect on breast health, especially the pain and discomfort associated with breast tenderness and lumps. In addition, caffeine inhibits the absorption of many nutrients and causes excessive loss of calcium, potassium, iron, magnesium, and trace minerals in the urine. This is particularly important for women, because loss of these essential minerals increases the chance of getting osteoporosis. Caffeine also raises the body's level of homocysteine, a compound which, at high levels, can cause heart attack, osteoporosis, and stroke. If you want to reduce or eliminate your intake of caffeine, refer to the recommendations in Chapter 4.

Alcohol

To drink or not to drink is a question that baffles many women. On the one hand, scientists say that having one alcoholic drink per day reduces a woman's risk of coronary artery disease, yet on the other hand, it increases her chances of getting breast cancer. Or does it? Must women decide if they can drink based on their personal risk of a specific disease? Researchers have not yet found definitive answers, but here is what is known so far.

What the Studies Show

The role of alcohol in causing or contributing to breast cancer has been the subject of many scientific studies. The risk appears to be real, although experts cannot seem to agree on the magnitude of that risk:

- In 1987, a *New England Journal of Medicine* article noted a 40 to 60% increase in breast cancer among women who drank moderately. A year later, Harvard University researchers reported that two drinks a day increased breast cancer risk by as much as 70% compared with nondrinkers.

- In 1993, researchers at the National Institute of Environmental Health Sciences discovered that when compared with women who did not drink alcohol, those who had one drink per day increased their breast cancer risk by 10%; those who had two drinks, 20%.

- A *Lancet* article published a few years later claimed alcohol consumption during the teenage years had the most significant impact on increasing a woman's risk of breast cancer.

- A 1997 National Cancer Institute study reported that drinking alcohol increased the risk of breast cancer among women younger than 45 years, and that it had a significant effect on women who had advanced breast cancer. However, the researchers contradicted earlier findings when it stated that "breast cancer risk was not influenced by drinking during the teenage years or early adulthood."

- A 1998 study looked at more than 322,000 women over 11 years. This study concluded that "among women who consume alcohol regularly, reducing alcohol consumption is a potential means to reduce breast cancer risk."

- In the Framingham study, more than 5000 women were followed for up to 40 years, and the researchers concluded that "the light consumption of alcohol or any type of alcoholic beverage is not associated with increased breast cancer risk."

- According to an April 1999 report by researchers at the National Institute of Environmental Health Sciences, "because of the modest association between alcohol and breast cancer and the generally moderate level of alcohol intake among U.S. women, the proportion of breast cancer attributable to alcohol intake is small."

The Bottom Line

When you look at all of the studies, one thing stands out: none of them say alcohol is not a risk, even if that risk is small. Thus, until more definitive data are gathered, most experts recommend avoiding alcohol, or, for women who believe they cannot give it up completely, seriously limiting intake to no more than two or three drinks per week.

Fat

Fat intake appears to be a significant risk factor for breast cancer. One of the first hints came in the 1950s, when researchers found that dietary fat promoted tumor growth in laboratory animals, particularly in the mammary glands. Since then, dozens of studies in humans make it clear that a high intake of dietary fat translates into a higher risk of breast cancer.

Revealing information was released in 1988, when the U.S. Surgeon General's Report showed that the countries with the highest intake of fat (especially found in meat and dairy) had the highest rates of breast cancer. Countries such as Japan, Thailand, Taiwan, and El Salvador, where the diet is largely plant based, have very low rates of breast cancer deaths, compared with countries where fat intake is high, such as the United States, Canada, the United Kingdom, and the Netherlands.

Since these results were released, there has been an increase in the incidence of breast cancer in Japan, the Philippines, and China. The introduction of the high-fat, low-fiber, animal-based Western diet to these countries, particularly fast food, has dramatically changed the cancer picture. Between 1970 and 1985, the incidence of breast cancer in Japan more than doubled. This bad luck has followed immigrants from these countries. Japanese, Filipino, and Chinese women who migrate to the United States and adopt the American diet now have the same high risk for breast cancer as their American peers.

The Controversy

When the results of the Harvard Nurses' Study were released in 1992, many people were surprised. It claimed that there was no relationship between fat intake and risk of breast cancer. This study has been criticized because it compared high-fat diets (ranging from 23% to 49%) and did not consider much lower fat intake, which many experts say is associated with lower rates of breast cancer. In fact, previous studies have indicated that fat intake must be 20% of calories or less to protect against cancer.

Even the National Academy of Sciences believes, "The scientific data do not provide a strong basis for establishing fat intake at precisely 30 percent of total calories. Indeed, the data could be used to justify an even greater reduction."

Udo Erasmus, Ph.D., author of *Fats That Heal, Fats That Kill*, and an internationally recognized expert on fats and human nutrition, joins the ranks of many other health care professionals, including John McDougall, M.D.; Dean Ornish, M.D.; Neal Barnard, M.D.; and the Physicians Committee for Responsible Medicine, in recommending that fat intake be 20% or lower of daily caloric intake. Although many find Dr. Ornish's regimen of 10% fat to be too strict (but effective in the treatment of heart disease), the consensus among many experts seems to be that 15 to 20% is a healthy and easily achievable range for cancer prevention and overall health.

In the hope that the controversy over the role of fat in breast cancer can be resolved, two major studies have been initiated. The Women's Health Initiative, sponsored by the National Institutes of Health, is investigating whether a low-fat diet (20% fat) can prevent breast cancer, colon cancer, and heart disease. Results will be available in 2005. The other study, sponsored by the National Cancer Institute and conducted by the American Health Foundation, is investigating whether a 15% fat intake benefits women who already have breast cancer. Results are expected in 2002.

Good Fat and Bad Fat

To familiarize yourself with the good and bad fats, read the following descriptions:

* *Saturated fats:* These "bad" fats are solid at room temperature. They are found mostly in animal foods (meats, poultry, dairy products) and in some vegetable products, such as coconut oil, palm kernel oil, and vegetable shortening. Saturated fat is associated with an increased risk of breast cancer, as well as many other cancers and diseases. The liver

uses saturated fats to manufacture cholesterol, so it's important to restrict intake of saturated fat for this reason as well. Saturated fats should make up less than 10% of your total fat intake.

- *Trans-fatty acids:* These unnatural fats are created through a process called hydrogenation, which transforms unsaturated fats into saturated fats. But you won't see the words "trans-fatty acids" on food labels. Instead, look for "hydrogenated" or "partially hydrogenated" oil among the ingredients. Margarine, shortening, crackers, baked goods, and junk foods are typically high in hydrogenated oils. Trans-fatty acids extend the shelf life of products, but they do nothing to extend the life of the people who eat them. In fact, trans-fatty acids appear to play a role in causing breast cancer. They also interfere with the body's ability to utilize the good essential fatty acids, raise the level of bad cholesterol, and lower the level of good cholesterol.

- *Polyunsaturated fats:* This group contains omega-3 and omega-6 fatty acids, which have both good and bad qualities. The omega-3s (also called linolenic oils) are found in flaxseed, hemp seed, walnut oils, and cold-water fish, such as salmon, tuna, and herring. Omega-3s protect against cancer and cardiovascular disease. Omega-6 fatty acids (also called linolenic oil) are found in vegetable oils, such as corn, safflower, and sunflower oils. In small amounts they can lower total cholesterol levels, but in larger amounts they can lower levels of the "good" cholesterol (high-density lipoprotein cholesterol), and they are associated with an increased risk of cancer (see Chapter 4).

- *Monounsaturated fats:* This category includes the fats most often recognized as being healthy: olive oil, peanut oil, or any other fresh, unprocessed oil (see Chapter 4).

Any fats, even the healthy ones, can turn toxic if heated. Erasmus notes that "Frying once or twice won't kill us, but after ten, twenty, or thirty years of eating fried foods, our cells accumulate altered and toxic products for which they have not evolved efficient detoxifying mechanisms." In *Total Breast Health*, Robin Keuneke explains that untoasted sesame oil and olive oil are the most stable of the unsaturated oils and therefore may be heated more safely than other unsaturated oils, which include safflower, corn, and canola. These three commonly used oils are treated with sodium hydroxide and phosphoric acid, and are deodorized, bleached, and heated at high temperatures, all of which makes them unhealthy and likely to be carcinogenic.

Fat and Toxins

Dietary fat, especially animal fats, often contain pesticides, hormones, fungicides, and other carcinogens. Food animals are fed large amounts of dangerous chemicals to make them fatter faster. These chemicals accumulate in the animal's fat, then are ingested by people. Because these toxins have an affinity for fat, women's breasts are a prime gathering spot for them. Thus, animal fat carries a double danger for women.

Fat and Estrogen

Given the compelling evidence that heightened exposure to estrogen is associated with an increased risk of breast cancer (see Chapter 10), the link between high fat intake and breast cancer is even more convincing. Estrogen has an affinity for fat. As a woman's fat intake increases, so do her levels of estrogen.

Recent study findings illustrate this concept well. At the University of Southern California, reasearchers found that women's estrogen levels are lowered by up to 23% when their intake of dietary fat is lowered to 10 to 20% of their diet. Significant reductions in estrogen were also seen in diets that contained 18 to 25% of calories from fat.

Scientists have also looked at fat intake, estrogen levels, and incidence of breast cancer among women who eat either a vegetarian or a vegan diet (no animal products at all). Fat intake is typically much lower in these women, so you would expect to see lower estrogen levels as well. Research findings bear this out. One study of premenopausal vegetarians showed estrogen levels 23% lower than in nonvegetarians, while another study of postmenopausal vegans revealed that they had estrogen levels up to 40% lower.

Similarly, obesity is a risk factor for breast cancer, and overweight women have higher levels of estrogen than thinner women. That's because fat cells produce estrogen from the hormone androgen in the body. The higher the percentage of body fat, the greater the production of estrogen.

Some scientists say the relationship between dietary fat and breast cancer risk is so strong, if women reduced their fat intake by 50%, the risk of breast cancer could be lowered by about 250%. Tips on how you can greatly reduce your intake of bad fats and still eat foods you enjoy are offered in Chapter 4.

Food Additives

Beef, pork, chicken, lamb, eggs, milk, and other animal products are considered by many health experts to harm your health because they contain saturated fats and cholesterol (cancer and heart disease promoters); they are low or devoid of vitamins and minerals (cancer protectors); and they have no fiber or phytochemicals (also cancer protectors). But there is another reason to avoid animal products: they contain carcinogenic elements such as pesticides, antibiotics, steroids, and other chemicals. And these substances are added intentionally.

Treated Meat

Between 1947 and 1983, U.S. beef producers routinely administered a known carcinogen to their cattle. Diethylstilbestrol, or DES, is a highly potent synthetic estrogenic chemical that speeds up the fattening process. Even after DES was shown to increase rates of breast and vaginal cancers in females and to cause a higher rate of urinary tract and reproductive abnormalities in males, use of DES continued until 1979, when the FDA banned it.

Yet producers continued to use DES illegally until 1983, when they switched to natural sex hormones such as progesterone, testosterone, and progestins, or their synthetic equals. But the switch did not come soon enough for about 3000 children and infants in the United States and Puerto Rico who had premature sexual development and ovarian cysts associated with hormone use in meat.

It is now feared that residual hormones in beef are causing other problems. According to results of a national survey published in 1997 in *Pediatrics*, 1% of white girls and 3% of black girls show signs of breast and/or pubic hair development by the age of 3. This is a far cry from the normal age of 10 to 12. High levels of hormones in meat and dairy products is one reason for this unusual occurrence, say some experts. In *The Breast Cancer Prevention Program*, Dr. Samuel Epstein and David Steinman note that "the extent to which hormonal meat contributes to increased breast cancer rates, apart from cancer of the uterus, prostate, and testis, has been virtually ignored." They warn that treated beef "may also have other endocrine-disruptive effects, such as hastening menarche," which is already occurring in the United States.

Switching to chicken won't save you from contamination. In addition to the bacteria salmonella and campylobacter, which cause food poisoning, chicken contains the carcinogen dioxin, which is allowed by the FDA. Other substances added to chicken feed include nitrofurans, which are possible carcinogens, and gentian violet, which is a known human carcinogen.

Contaminated Dairy Products

While beef is contaminated with sex hormones, dairy cattle are treated with a genetically engineered product called recombinant bovine growth hormone, or rBGH, which affects milk products. This synthetic hormone increases milk production by about 10%. But it also causes an udder infection in cows called mastitis, which contaminates the milk with pus and bacteria. Infected cows must be treated with antibiotics, and these drugs can then contaminate the milk and may be linked with antibiotic-resistant infections in humans.

Giving rBGH to cows also causes their milk to be contaminated with insulin-like growth factor I (IGF-I). A link between elevated levels of IGF-I and breast cancer was suggested by Dr. Samuel Epstein in 1990, and his findings were supported by Dr. Susan Hankinson in 1998, who found a 700% increased risk of breast cancer among premenopausal women who had the highest levels of IGF-I in their blood. In addition, several studies in the *International Journal of Health Services* report a link between high levels of IGF-I in dairy products and risk of breast cancer.

Smoking

It's a given that smoking is bad for your health, but is it specifically harmful for your breasts? At first, a Canadian study conducted between 1982 and 1985 seemed to indicate that it was not. Investigators said their data "showed no evidence of an elevated risk [of breast cancer] for women with a history of cigarette smoking" or "of elevated risk in ex-smokers or current smokers."

But these findings were quickly disputed. The American Cancer Society (ACS) studied more than a half-million cancer-free women for more than 6 years. The ACS report in 1994 noted that women who smoked were 25% more likely to die of breast cancer than nonsmokers or ex-smokers. A woman's chance of dying of breast cancer increased proportionately as the number of cigarettes she smoked daily increased. The ACS researchers concluded that smoking lowers women's immune response, especially the number of natural killer cells, and thus smokers are less able to fight off the cancer.

Then in 1996, Swiss researchers suggested what was at the time a revolutionary concept: that passive tobacco smoke exposure triples the risk of getting breast cancer. Among smokers in their study, women who smoked more than a pack a day had a 4.6-fold risk of breast cancer.

Little research has focused on the effects of smoking on benign breast conditions. A 1999 Canadian study looked for an association between cigarette smoking and the risk of benign proliferative epithelial disorders of the breast (BPED) among 56,837 women. In these disorders, cells multiply beyond what is considered to be normal (proliferative). Sometimes the cells are abnormal, in which case experts believe there may be an increased risk of breast cancer. The researchers did not find a relationship between cigarette smoking and BPED. However, there are still good reasons not to smoke.

Sugar and Artificial Sweeteners

It's hard to believe there could be a link between sugar and breast cancer, but a few researchers seem to think there is one. In 1983, two researchers saw a possible connection and published their findings in *Medical Hypothesis*. After that time, interest seemed to fade.

But then in 1998, Dr. V. J. Burley at the University of Leeds, United Kingdom, analyzed all the available research on sugar and cancer and determined that "There is some suggestion of a weak increase in risk of breast cancer with high consumption of sucrose-containing foods." Such foods, which include cakes and other baked goods, also typically contain saturated fat, which is also implicated in breast cancer. Thus, Dr. Burley concluded that "It is apparent that there is insufficient evidence to conclude whether sugar has a role in cancer."

Artificial Sweeteners

Although there are no human studies that definitively link artificial sweeteners with breast cancer, research in laboratory animals has shown a relationship between intake of aspartame (in NutraSweet and Equal) and the development of breast tumors. In humans, artificial sweeteners such as aspartame and saccharin can cause headache, dizziness, dry eyes, memory loss, depression, mood swings, and gastrointestinal problems.

Environmental Toxins and Breast Cancer

In 1962, publication of *Silent Spring* by Rachel Carson brought to the public's attention the potential cancer-causing effects of an environmental pollutant known as DDT (chloropheno-thane). This pesticide, classified as an organochlorine, was once used widely in the United States in agriculture. Carson's work and that of many of her peers prompted the U.S. government in the 1970s to ban the use of DDT and PCBs (polychlorinated biphenyls), another group of carcinogenic chemicals. Unfortunately, these chemicals still linger in the water and soil and are still found in some foods; and many foreign countries use these chemicals on crops exported to the United States.

During the nearly four decades since Carson's discovery, many studies have shown a connection between organochlorine use and breast cancer. In 1992, for example, Dr. Frank Falck Jr. found that women with breast cancer had higher levels of organochlorines in their fatty breast tissue than did women without breast cancer. In 1993, Dr. Mary Wolff of Mount Sinai School of Medicine in New York analyzed the blood samples of women with and without breast cancer and found that those with cancer had significantly higher levels of DDE (a derivative of DDT). In fact, the women with high levels of DDE were four times more likely to have breast cancer than those who had low levels.

Frightening news was released in 1994, when a New York State Department of Health report announced that women who lived near any of several chemical plants on Long Island,

New York, for at least 10 years had a 60% greater chance of having breast cancer after menopause than women in the general population. If this is true of women who live near these plants, what about the people who work in them?

There are many cases of high rates of cancer and other diseases being linked with workplace pollutants; for example, asbestos, coal tars, and radon are associated with various lung diseases. It is likely only a matter of time before the health risks of organochlorines and other chemicals are linked with breast cancer and other diseases.

Contradictory Findings

Just when a connection between organocholorines and breast cancer seemed clear, Dr. Nancy Krieger uncovered different results. Her 1994 study, published in the *Journal of the National Cancer Institute*, found no significant connection between increased risk of breast cancer and increased levels of DDE among white women, a borderline significance among black women, and no significance between decreased risk of breast cancer and increased DDE among Asian women.

Environmental Factors and Estrogens

Had scientists been wrong all those years? Many don't think so. What a growing number do believe, however, is that they need to investigate a theory: that the chance of developing breast cancer increases with a woman's lifetime exposure to estrogen. That is, the longer estrogen circulates through a woman's body, and the greater levels of the hormone she has, the greater her chances of getting breast cancer. Researchers have been following this concept for many years, but not until recently did they consider it in the context of pesticides and other environmental factors. Their studies involve a different type of estrogen—chemical compounds that come from the environment and act like estrogens—called xenoestrogens.

Xenoestrogens: The "Bad" Estrogens

Researchers have overwhelming evidence that estrogen is intimately connected with the development of breast cancer (see Chapter 10). Therefore, the discovery that organochlorine pesticides and other common products in the environment contain xenoestrogens cast a new light on the link between these possible carcinogens and breast cancer. (Don't confuse xenoestrogens with *phytoestrogens*, the "good" estrogens found in plants. They are discussed in Chapter 4.)

Although xenoestrogens have a different chemical structure than the natural estrogen your body produces, they can trigger potentially harmful estrogenic activity in the body. Xenoestrogens enter the body through the skin, in food and water, and in the air. They are found in pesticides, herbicides, lubricated condoms, cosmetics, hair dyes, detergents, synthetic leather, the lining of food cans, and plastic food wraps.

Xenoestrogens Are All Around You

There are probably dozens of potentially cancer-causing products in your home right now. When considered individually, your exposure to these items probably doesn't pose a great cancer risk, but experts warn that the damage they cause builds up gradually.

Take, for instance, canned foods. In 1988, two researchers at the Tufts University School of Medicine discovered that xenoestrogens in plastic-coated food cans can leak into the food. In *The Truth About Breast Cancer*, author Joseph Keon, Ph.D., recommends that women avoid products in plastic bottles with the number 3 on the bottom, because the vinyl chloride can seep into foods and beverages.

Dr. Keon and other experts also advise against using clingy plastic wraps, such as those used to wrap meat and cheese, and the rolls you can purchase for home use, because they are made with a chemical called di-(2-ethylhexyl)adipate, also known as DEHA. (Do not confuse this with DHEA, a hormone precursor.) Animal studies suggest that DEHA can interfere with hormone activity and possibly cause breast cancer, birth defects, low sperm levels, and mental problems.

The Consumers Union tested both commercial and retail brands of plastic cling wrap and found that the brands used by supermarkets contain high levels of DEHA, whereas most retail brands such as Saran Wrap and Glad are DEHA-free. One retail brand, Reynolds Plastic Wrap, contains some DEHA. To protect yourself against the possibility of DEHA contamination, you can do the following:

- Avoid foods that are encased in cling wrap. If you have a choice, ask for paper instead.
- If the product is wrapped, remove the plastic when you get home and store the food in another container.
- Do not use plastic wrap to cover food when heating or cooking in the microwave.

Protect Yourself Against Common Carcinogens

Some other common household products that contain carcinogens are listed below. Chronic exposure to these substances may increase your risk of breast cancer:

- No-pest strips and pest sprays that contain DDVP (dichlorvos), which the Environmental Protection Agency has linked with "an unacceptably high risk of cancer in people and pets."
- Spray paint and aerosol strippers that contain methylene chloride.
- Lawn and home pesticides that contain atrazine.
- Kerosene heaters and gas burners, which emit 1,8-dinitropyrene, benzopyrene, and 2-nitrofluorene.
- Natural gas heating and cooking appliances, which emit benzene.
- Permanent and semipermanent hair dyes: many contaminants, including paraphenylenediamine, formaldehyde-

releasing preservatives, and dioxane. Several studies link long-term hair dye use with breast cancer.

* Bleach, ammonia, oven cleaners, spot removers, paints, disinfectants, home foggers, and adhesive cements, all of which contain highly volatile chemicals that are easily inhaled.

Other Considerations

At the Mount Sinai School of Medicine in New York City, Drs. Wolff and Weston believe that one reason clearly defined links between environmental contaminants and breast cancer are difficult to establish is that other factors need to be looked at as well. These include the fact that scientists don't fully understand tumor development, and that genes can influence the metabolism of environmental contaminants. Timing also plays a critical part. A woman's age and whether she is pre-menopausal, pregnant, or postmenopausal, appear to have an effect on susceptibility to cancer-causing agents.

Pesticides and Food: Your Poisoned Plate

According to the National Resources Defense Council, 845 million pounds of poisonous chemicals were applied to American crops in 1997. The Environmental Protection Agency (EPA) reports that 90% of all fungicides, 60% of all herbicides, and 30% of all insecticides are carcinogenic. The National Academy of Sciences reports that pesticide use might be responsible for an additional 1.4 million cases of cancer among Americans, as well as cause nerve damage, birth defects, and genetic mutations. Among this pesticide use, more than 2 million pounds of endosulfan are used on U.S. crops such as lettuce, carrots, tomatoes, and spinach. Endosulfan, along with two other widely used pesticides, methoxychlor and dicofol, have estrogen-like effects, and, like DDT, have the potential to cause breast cancer.

Not everyone agrees that pesticides pose a great cancer risk. American Institute for Cancer Research (AICR) president Marilyn Gentry emphasizes that cancer is preventable, and that preventing cancer doesn't involve avoiding potential carcinogens as much as it does making healthy changes in lifestyle, including eating lots of fruits and vegetables, and getting routine exercise. Although many people agree that a healthy lifestyle is of major importance in preventing cancer, they also firmly believe that pesticide use is a real danger and that organic foods are their safest hedge against cancer when it comes to food choices. Results of an AICR survey found that 77% of American adults believe they can reduce their risk of cancer by not eating produce that has been sprayed with pesticides. For many people, any risk of cancer from pesticides is enough reason to avoid them.

While the AICR study recommends increasing intake of fruits and vegetables, it strongly discourages meat consumption. Food animals are prime reservoirs for pesticides and other chemicals that seep into the soil and water, which are then consumed by animals. These toxins, along with hormones, steroids, and other drugs given to food animals, collect in the animals' fat. The AICR recommends eating organic meat only, and no more than once a week.

Radiation

High-level radiation, whether it is in the form of chest or dental x-rays or the explosion of an atomic bomb, has been linked with breast cancer. (Even low- and mid-level radiation, such as that emitted by televisions [low] and microwaves [mid], is considered to be cancer-causing by some individuals.) Radiation at the high end of the energy spectrum can destroy the chemical makeup of living organisms and produce body-damaging substances called free radicals. These free radicals have the ability to produce cancer.

Radiation and Breast Cancer

One of the first hints that radiation causes breast cancer came when researchers noted high rates of the disease among women who had survived the bombings of Nagasaki and Hiroshima. More links have been found in cases where radiation is used to heal or diagnose rather than harm. In 1971, investigators noted high rates of breast cancer among adults who as infants had received radiation treatments for an enlarged thymus gland. Another study found increased cancer rates among adults who had been exposed to 100 or more x-rays as children when they were monitored for tuberculosis. Unfortunately, physicians in the early twentieth century unknowingly subjected tens of thousands of children to excessive radiation to either treat or diagnose medical conditions, including curvature of the spine, Hodgkin's disease, infected nipples and breasts (mastitis), fungal scalp infections, and acne.

Excessive exposure to radiation continues today. Women who undergo fluoroscopy, such as barium enemas, barium swallows, or cardiac catheterization, are exposed to high doses of radiation. Dentists, orthopedists, and pulmonologists also use x-rays. Although the breast is not directly radiated in most of these cases, the body still receives the damaging effects. If you are at risk for breast cancer, discuss your concerns with your doctor or dentist and ask if the x-rays are absolutely necessary.

Generally, experts believe that the amount of radiation women receive from a mammogram after age 40 is safe. However, because younger women are generally more susceptible to radiation, regular mammograms in younger women are not recommended.

Radiation, Genes, and Hormones

Up to 2% of women carry a gene for ataxia-telangiectasia (A-T), an uncommon genetic disease that causes progressive neurological problems and skin lesions. Women with A-T are highly susceptible to the carcinogenic effects of radiation and have a 5-fold increased risk for developing breast cancer.

These women are in a difficult situation: Because they are at high risk of breast cancer, doctors recommend routine mammograms beginning at an early age, yet those same mammograms expose them to a greater risk of cancer.

Other women who are unusually sensitive to the damaging effects of radiation are those who have high levels of total estrogen. This category includes women who have never had children or who have had children late in life. It has been proposed that women who take hormonal contraceptives or estrogen replacement therapy or who eat animal foods that are contaminated with estrogens may also be at higher risk of breast cancer from radiation.

Electromagnetic Fields

The word *electromagnetic* describes the partnership of electric and magnetic fields. Electrical fields are characterized by charged particles called ions, and magnetic fields involve the movement of ions as they travel through an electric current. The difference between these two fields is that electricity stays within its circuitry while magnetic fields break out and penetrate everything in their path, including people. So when you turn on your hair dryer, electricity surges through the cord and magnetic energy flies out of the dryer.

The magnetic energy coming from appliances is minuscule compared with the amount that emanates from high-voltage lines that crisscross the United States. These high-current lines became cancer suspects in 1979, when two researchers noted that there were a high number of cancer deaths in Denver among young children who lived near high-voltage lines.

Electromagnetic Fields and Breast Cancer
In 1987, Drs. Nancy Wertheimer and Edward Leeper found increased rates of breast cancer among premenopausal women living near electrical transmission lines in Colorado. Although most of the work focused on brain and blood cancer (leukemia), breast cancer entered the picture in 1991 when three different

investigations found high rates of breast cancer among male electrical employees. Soon afterward, Dr. Dana Loomis of the University of North Carolina found a 38% higher rate of death from breast cancer among women electrical workers than among female nonelectrical workers. In yet another study, scientists found a link between breast cancer and women who worked as telephone repairers, line workers, or installers.

But researchers cannot explain how electromagnetic fields (EMFs) cause breast cancer. One popular theory is that EMFs suppress the body's release of melatonin, a hormone produced by the pineal gland, which inhibits the production of estrogen. If melatonin levels are low, estrogen levels can rise, and elevated estrogen levels are associated with cancer growth (see Chapter 11). To study the link between EMFs and breast cancer, scientists looked at the effects of EMFs on breast cancer cells and animals with breast cancer. They exposed half of a group of female rats with breast cancer to 60 hertz power, which is the power used in the United States. The exposed rats developed 50% more cancerous tumors than the control rats.

The Debate

Not every study has had the same results, however. At the National Institute of Environmental Health Sciences in North Carolina, Dr. G. A. Boorman exposed rats to 13 and 26 weeks of electromagnetic energy and did not see a significant cancerous effect. In 1996, the American Cancer Society claimed that "no form of electromagnetic energy at frequency levels below those of ionizing radiation (x-rays) and ultraviolet radiation has been shown to cause cancer." And in 1999, a *Carcinogenesis* article stated that "EMF is unlikely to influence breast cancer induction through a mechanism involving altered expression of genes."

Some people disagree, including the EMR Alliance, an organization that represents U.S. citizen groups. They point to cases such as those mentioned above, and a 1991 study from the Boston University School of Public Health, in which an increased risk of breast cancer was found among women who lived within 500 feet of electric power substations in Cape Cod, Massachusetts. And so the debate continues.

At Risk on the Job

You may be getting more from your job than a paycheck. Scientists have identified more than fifty occupational cancer-causing substances that have induced breast cancer in laboratory animals. Researchers believe these compounds will have the same effect on women who are exposed to these toxins in their workplace.

Scientists have identified four of the primary carcinogens used in the workplace: benzene, methylene chloride (dichloromethane), ethylene oxide, and phenylenediamine dyes. Approximately one million women work in the petrochemical, cosmetology, or manufacturing industries and are exposed to these toxins. Another cancer risk, radiation, affects many health care professionals.

- Cosmetologists: Studies from the late 1950s up to 1993 show an excessive amount of breast cancer among hairdressers. The link appears to be the use of hair dyes, which have induced breast cancer in laboratory animals.

- Pharmaceutical workers: Researchers believe it is the workers' chronic exposure to estrogens and progestins that place them at high risk for breast cancer.

- Artists (painters): Artists who paint with oils may be exposed to an excessive amount of carcinogens, including benzene and methylene chloride.

- Radiation workers: Individuals who do diagnostic x-rays for medical or dental professionals have the potential to be exposed to excessive amounts of radiation. Evidence of the association between radiation and breast cancer is supported by animal studies, by studies in women who survived the atom bomb, and by those who have received therapeutic radiation.

The American Cancer Society and several public health organizations have conducted studies to determine if there is an increased risk of breast cancer associated with certain occupations. In 1982, the American Cancer Society began a study in which investigators observed 563,395 women free of cancer and followed them for 9 years. When the deaths from breast cancer of 1780 women were examined, researchers found only a slightly increased risk among women in administrative support and managerial positions, but none among teachers, librarians, service workers, housewives, or nurses. Similar results were found in a study done by the Boston University School of Public Health, published in 1996.

Exposure to some of the substances that compromise your breast health are beyond your control, but others are not. You can choose to use or avoid fats, nicotine, sugar, caffeine, and food additives and select healthy alternatives.

The influx of unnatural, manmade chemicals into our food and environment has a negative impact on our health and our planet. Be cautious about such products, learn all you can about them, and then make an informed decision about whether you will expose yourself to them. Although no one factor alone may cause cancer, several factors together, over time, appear to be hazardous. Just as there are many causes of cancer, there are many ways to prevent it. When you eliminate pesticides from your garden, refuse to use plastic wrap, choose organic rather than conventionally grown foods, and avoid unnecessary x-rays, you enhance your health rather than compromise it.

C H A P T E R   T E N

※

Breast Cancer

No woman ever wants to hear these words: "You have breast cancer." Yet every year, 180,000 women in the United States will hear them. Breast cancer is the most common cancer that affects women in the United States, and it is the leading cause of cancer deaths in women. If you thought we were winning the war against cancer, think again: the Centers for Disease Control reports that the incidence of breast cancer increased 52% between 1950 and 1990. Every 11 minutes a woman loses her battle with it.

But you can fight back. In fact, the information in this book gives you the tools to do so. This chapter presents the nuts and bolts of breast cancer so that you can become better acquainted with what you're fighting. Included is concise, easy-to-understand information about the risk factors, methods of diagnosis, stages of development, and conventional treatments (including surgery, radiation, chemotherapy, and hormone treatment), plus the latest studies. This chapter can help you, along with your health care provider, to take informed steps in the prevention and treatment of breast cancer. While conventional treatment options are explained here, you are referred to Chapters 4, 5, and 7 for natural ways to complement your treatment plan.

What Is Cancer?

Cancer is the uncontrolled reproduction or growth of cells that have been damaged. The damage occurs when a carcinogen, like those discussed in Chapter 9, affects an area within the nucleus of the cell called the proto-oncogene (*onco* comes from the Greek word *onkos*, which means "tumor" or "bump"), a gene that controls cell growth and multiplication. Once the gene has been affected, every offspring cell carries the damaged oncogene, and the spread of cancer begins.

Cancer cells divide faster than normal cells, and this ability allows them to take over areas once occupied by healthy cells and to cause additional damage to tissue, bone, and nerves. In breast cancer, the growth usually begins in the drainage ducts of the mammary glands.

What Is Breast Cancer?

Experts believe breast cancer develops as epithelial cells that line the ducts in the breast become damaged and begin an abnormal growth process, called hyperplasia. This results in a cluster of atypical cells—cells that are different from normal breast cells but are not necessarily cancerous. If these cells are prompted into an uncontrollable growth stage, the process of breast cancer has begun.

At first, breast cancer cells develop inside the breast ducts. This type of cancer is called intraductal (or ductal) carcinoma in situ, which means it is contained in the duct (intraductal) and has not spread outside (in situ) the duct lining. These cancers are typically less than 1 centimeter (less than ½ inch) in diameter and rarely cause a lump or thickening. Because they are too soft and small to detect using physical examination, mammography is usually needed. The mammogram typically shows flecks of calcium, called microcalcifications, which look like grains of sand. Microcalcifications occur when calcium salts get deposited in dead cells. Approximately 15 to 20% of all breast cancers diagnosed are intraductal carcinoma in situ.

If these cancer cells are not detected, they eventually break through the outer lining of the ducts and begin to invade the breast and surrounding tissues. At this point, the cancer is *invasive*, and it is commonly known as ductal carcinoma. Ductal carcinoma accounts for 70 to 80% of all detected breast cancer.

Once the breast cancer cells become invasive, the lymph vessels can transport them to the lymph nodes that surround the breast and those under the breastbone and in the armpit. These cells are sometimes carried to other parts of the body. This process is called metastasis. You may hear about a breast cancer that has metastasized, which means the breast cancer cells have invaded other areas.

A small percentage of breast cancers are found in the lobules of the breast. Lobular carcinoma in situ, sometimes called lobular neoplasia (new growth), involves abnormal cells that grow within the lobules, or milk-producing glands, but they do not extend beyond the lobule walls. There is some debate about this type of cancer. Some researchers say it does not become an invasive cancer but that women with lobular carcinoma in situ are at a greater risk of developing an invasive breast cancer elsewhere in the same breast or in the other breast.

Diagnosing Breast Cancer

Breast cancer does not appear suddenly overnight. The cancer develops from extremely small cells and it may take up to 10 years or longer before the growth is large enough to be detected, either by palpation (feeling it) during a breast examination or through mammography (see Chapter 8 for details on these procedures).

The most common sign of breast cancer is a new mass or lump in the breast. If you do breast self-examination regularly, you will recognize a new lump because it will be different from the usual bumps you feel in your breasts. A breast cancer lump is typically painless and hard, and has irregular edges. In rare cases, they are soft, tender, and rounded. Therefore, to be safe, report any *unusual* lump to a health care provider who is an expert in breast disease. Other signs of breast cancer may include swelling of a part of the breast even without a detectable lump, an unusual discharge from the nipple, skin dimpling or irritation, rash or redness of the nipple or skin of the breast, or nipple pain. Rarely, enlarged lymph nodes under the arm are detected before a breast lump can be felt.

Screening for Breast Cancer

The first step in diagnosing breast cancer is screening for the disease. Breast self-examination, physical examination by a physician, and mammography are the three first-line screening methods for breast cancer and other breast problems. Details on all three procedures are covered in Chapter 8.

Mammography is the subject of considerable debate, particularly concerning its safety and the need for regular mammograms. There is also great concern over the message women get that mammograms and physical examinations are important in preventing breast cancer. The truth is, neither method *prevents* breast cancer—they can only detect it. Preventive measures include making healthy lifestyle choices and avoiding carcinogens. Yet many physicians fail to stress these preventive actions. They also neglect to mention that there are other diagnostic screening approaches, such as magnetic resonance imaging and positron emission tomography, that women can access if they want to avoid mammograms. Some of these alternatives are explained in Chapter 8.

What Happens If I Find a Lump?

If you or your physician find a lump during a physical examination, a mammogram will be taken. If the mammogram shows that the area of abnormal tissue (lesion) is not cancerous, you can return to your routine examination schedule. If the lesion is suspicious, the doctor may take a special image called a *cone view with magnification*, which makes it easier to evaluate the area in question. If the abnormal area appears to be benign (not cancerous), you will probably be asked to come back in 3 to 6 months to have another mammogram. Finally, the physician may decide to do a biopsy to determine if the lesion is indeed cancer.

Biopsy

Every year, more than one million women undergo a breast biopsy. For now, this is the only way to determine if an abnormal growth is cancerous. A biopsy is a tissue sample that is examined under a microscope. The sample can be obtained in a few different ways, and your physician should consult with you about the method he or she thinks is best, including the advantages and disadvantages of each. Factors to be considered when choosing a biopsy approach are your general state of health and the size, location, and number of lesions.

Fine-needle aspiration biopsy involves placing a needle into the area in question while the doctor palpates (feels) the lump. If the lump is difficult to locate, the doctor may use ultrasound to guide the needle to the site. Once the needle enters the lump, fluid is withdrawn, or, in the absence of fluid, tiny tissue fragments. If the fluid is clear, the lump is most likely a benign cyst. Cloudy or bloody fluid is found in benign cysts, also, although in rare cases the growth is cancerous. If the lump is solid or semisolid and tissue fragments are taken, they are examined to determine if the lump is benign or malignant.

If the results of the fine-needle biopsy are not conclusive, your physician will likely do another type of biopsy. If the fine-needle biopsy indicates a benign lump but your doctor is still suspicious, he or she may order a repeat biopsy or may ask you to come in for a follow-up physical examination and mammography in a few months.

If a *core-needle biopsy* is chosen, you will receive a local anesthetic before your doctor inserts a larger-bore needle into the abnormal breast tissue and obtains tissue samples about $\frac{1}{16}$ to $\frac{1}{8}$ inch in diameter and $\frac{1}{2}$ inch long. Three to five samples are usually collected.

A *surgical biopsy* is needed when the doctor believes it's necessary to remove all or part of the mass for examination. This procedure is usually done under local anesthesia and intravenous sedation at an outpatient facility. Most physicians do an excisional biopsy, in which the entire lesion plus some surrounding tissue is removed and examined. If the mass is benign, no treatment is needed. If it is malignant, the patient can take some time to gather information and make an informed decision about how to deal with her condition.

The Advanced Breast Biopsy Instrument, or ABBI, is a new approach to doing biopsy. The ABBI is less invasive than traditional biopsy, uses a local anesthetic, and makes a smaller incision; thus, it leaves a smaller scar ($\frac{1}{2}$ to 1 inch). The machine gives a three-dimensional view of where the lesion is located and allows for very accurate sample collection.

Ultrasound

Sometimes doctors order ultrasound, also known as sonography, which uses high-frequency sound waves to make an image of the abnormal tissue. This procedure does not involve radiation. Generally, ultrasound is used in the following situations:

- To determine whether a questionable area detected on a mammogram is a solid tumor or a fluid-filled cyst
- When there is an abnormality on a mammogram but no lump can be detected
- For women who have very dense breasts and a family history of breast cancer
- For pregnant or breast-feeding women with breast problems
- To detect an implant leak

In 1996, the Food and Drug Administration (FDA) approved the use of high-definition digital ultrasound for diagnosing questionable masses found during routine mammography. It is believed this procedure could reduce the number of breast biopsies in the United States by 40%. Ultrasound is not a substitute for mammography.

Tests for Nipple Discharge

Nipple discharge during a physical examination is normal in 50 to 60% of white women and black women, and 40% of Asian women. If you have nipple discharge, your physician may elect to do an x-ray called a ductogram. This procedure involves injecting contrast medium into the duct and then viewing the results to see if there is a mass inside the duct. Sometimes the discharged fluid is examined under a microscope for the presence of cancerous cells. If the secretions are milky or clear, chances are no cancer is present. If the discharge is red or brown, it usually indicates an infection or a benign tumor, although sometimes it indicates cancer.

Breast Biophysical Examination (BBE)

In July 1998, *The Lancet* published the results of a study in which researchers had tested a new noninvasive diagnostic technique for breast cancer. Called BBE, or Breast Biophysical Examination, it has been described as "an EKG [electrocardiogram] for the breast," according to Neil B. Friedman, M.D., director of the Breast Center at Mercy Medical Center. The BBE helps physicians distinguish benign masses from breast cancer. The best candidates for BBE are premenopausal women who have had an abnormality detected during clinical breast examination.

The test, which was developed by Biofield Corporation in Roswell, Georgia, records and analyzes changes in electrical charges that are painlessly applied to the breast. It has been very sensitive in identifying lesions, and it is hoped it will help eliminate thousands of unnecessary biopsies that are performed each year. Although it has been approved for use in Europe, FDA approval is still forthcoming in the United States.

Staging Breast Cancer

If breast cancer is diagnosed, the stage of disease needs to be determined. Staging is a classification method that helps physicians choose the best treatment. First, the cancer is classified as either invasive or noninvasive. Then it is graded from stage 0 to stage IV, with stage I being the preinvasive form. Up to 40% of women who do not get treated for Stage I develop invasive cancer. Each of the four stages has three elements: size of the tumor, extent of lymph node involvement, and extent of metastasis. Although there are several staging systems, most health care professionals use the Histopathologic TNM Classification (*T* for tumor, *N* for node, *M* for metastasis) prepared by the American Joint Committee on Cancer and the International Union Against Cancer (see below).

Breast Cancer Classifications

Stage 0   Ductal carcinoma in situ is the earliest form of breast cancer. Cancer cells are confined to a duct. Lobular carcinoma in situ is sometimes placed in this category.

Stage I   The tumor is less than 2 centimeters (about ¾ inch) in diameter and has not extended beyond the breast.

Stage II   Tumor size is greater than 2 centimeters and/or has spread to the lymph nodes under the arm on the same side as the breast cancer. At this stage, the malignant lymph nodes are not attached to the surrounding tissue or to one another.

Stage III   Tumor size is either greater than 5 centimeters (more than 2 inches) in diameter or has extended to lymph nodes that are attached to one another or to surrounding tissue. Also included in this stage are breast cancers of any size that have spread to the chest wall, the internal mammary lymph nodes, or the skin.

Stage IV   Breast cancer, regardless of size, that has metastasized to distant organs, bones, or lymph nodes not near the breast is included in stage IV.

Hormone Receptor Status

When a biopsy is done, your doctor will determine if hormone receptors are present. Normal breast cells and some breast cancer cells have receptors that recognize and attract estrogen and progesterone, hormones that play a critical part in the treatment and prognosis of breast cancer. Breast cancers that have these receptors are usually referred to as estrogen-receptor (ER)–positive and progesterone-receptor (PR)–positive tumors. The prognosis for ER-positive and PR-positive cancers is better than for negative tumors and more likely to respond to hormone therapy (see "Hormonal Therapy," later in this chapter).

Lymph Node Involvement

Invasive cancer often spreads to the lymph nodes, structures in the lymphatic system that filter harmful substances, such as bacteria and cancer cells, and thus enhance the immune system. The axillary, or armpit, lymph nodes are the ones most often involved in metastasized breast cancer. Occasionally, lymph nodes around the collarbone or behind the ribs are affected. If breast cancer has spread to the lymph nodes, chances that the cancer will metastasize to other parts of the body increase. The more nodes involved, the greater the risk.

Other Tests That Predict Prognosis

Ongoing breast cancer research is finding ways to more accurately determine prognosis. One way is with DNA (deoxyribonucleic acid) cytometry, which uses lasers and computers to identify the amount of DNA in cancer cells. Breast cancer cells with an abnormal amount of DNA are *aneupoid* and are believed to be more aggressive than cells with a normal amount of DNA, which are called *diploid*. Cytometry can also measure the percentage of cells in a given sample that are in a specific stage of cell division called the *synthesis* phase. The more cells in this phase, the more aggressive the cancer is likely to be.

Other new tests include those that look at changes in a tumor suppressor gene known as p53 or in the epidermal growth factor receptor. Yet another test determines the density of the small blood vessels that supply nutrients to cancer cells. All of these tests can help physicians determine which type of treatment is best for a given patient.

Risk Factors for Breast Cancer

Age

The largest number of breast cancers occur in women between the ages of 50 and 70. One-third of all cases affect women younger than 50, and 18% are found in women in their 40s. Breast cancer in women younger than 30 is unusual. But since the mid-1980s, the breast cancer rate among all age groups has been increasing. Experts say the rise is not related to the greater use of mammography, but may be associated with environmental toxins, delayed childbearing, dietary fat, or other causes.

Race

White women are at greater risk of breast cancer than women of other racial groups. Mortality, however, is a different matter. A report in the January 2000 issue of *Cancer* shows that black women are 67% more likely to die of breast cancer than white women. The researchers propose that economic, genetic, and cultural factors are to blame. Black women are more likely to get breast cancer at an earlier age, and such breast cancer is typically more aggressive than disease that occurs later in life. Thus, the investigators suggest that black women begin mammogram screening before age 40 in the hope that cancer will be detected and treated at an earlier stage. There is a greater prevalence of obesity among black women and possibly a greater fear of radiation treatment, which may be responsible for the higher death rate from breast cancer.

Genetics

Many people are under the impression that genetics is a big risk factor for breast cancer. In reality, only about 6 to 10% of breast cancer incidence is attributed to a genetic predisposition. This is important to remember in light of the information about breast cancer genes that has recently become the subject of much research and debate.

Research into the genetics of breast cancer is uncovering critical information about how the disease may be inherited. Several breast cancer genes have been identified and labeled as BRCA1 and BRCA2 (breast cancer 1 and 2). When these genes undergo a change or mutation, the result is an increased chance of developing breast cancer. The type of mutation that occurs determines the percentage of increased risk, as well as whether there is an associated risk of another type of cancer.

So far scientists have identified more than 100 types of mutations, so the possibility of different kinds of cancer is great. For example, mutation of both genes is associated with an increased breast cancer risk of 50 to 75% over a lifetime, while mutation of only one gene lowers the risk. Both genes have also been linked with an increased risk of ovarian cancer, but only BRCA2 is associated with male breast cancer. A third gene, called TSG101, is associated with suppression of tumor development. Some women with breast cancer either do not have this gene or it is damaged.

Along with the discovery of BRCA1 and BRCA2 has come a test that enables women to learn if they have these breast cancer genes. Many doctors are against offering this test, and many women are equally if not more concerned. One question that arises is what to do with the information. If a woman learns that she has the breast cancer genes, it does not guarantee she will get breast cancer. Some argue that knowing will allow women to take all the preventive measures they can (eating healthy, avoiding carcinogens, and so on), while others counter that women in high-risk groups would be the ones opting for the test, and so they should be taking precautions anyway.

But an even bigger concern may be the effect a positive test result can have on women's chances of getting or keeping their health insurance or their job, and the psychological impact on them and their family. There is also the chance that the test results may give a false positive (saying the genes are present when they are not) and upset women unnecessarily, or even worse. Every year thousands of women who are at high risk of developing breast cancer undergo preventive mastectomy. The removal of one or both healthy breasts as a means to prevent what these women believe is an inevitable diagnosis of cancer could be a consequence of women learning they have the cancer genes. Thus, experts strongly urge any woman who is interested in the breast cancer genetic test to undergo extensive counseling with a genetic counselor.

Family History

A woman's family history of breast cancer is an indicator of whether she will develop the same disease. Surprisingly, a woman has a greater chance of getting breast cancer if her sister developed the disease than if her mother did. A woman whose sister developed breast cancer has a 2.5 times greater risk of getting the disease herself than if her sister were cancer-free. That same woman has a 2-fold increased risk of getting breast cancer if her mother's cancer occurred before the age of 40. For women who have a brother who has prostate cancer, their chance of getting breast cancer is increased 4-fold. Study results published by the Mayo Clinic in February 2000 show that fraternal twin sisters are twice as likely to get breast cancer after menopause than women who are not twins. The theory is that there are intrauterine influences on cancer of the breast, but they are currently unknown.

Early Menstruation

Females who get their first period before age 13 have a 4.2 times greater risk of developing breast cancer than those who first menstruate at a later age. The reason has to do with estrogen levels. The earlier menstruation begins, the more periods a woman will have over her lifetime, which increases the amount of estrogen that will flow through her body. Although a few extra years of exposure to estrogen may not seem like a lot, a young woman's breast tissue is especially susceptible to estrogen exposure during the teen years.

Although adult women can do nothing to change this risk for themselves, they can help influence when menarche begins for their daughters and nieces. Early menarche is associated with the increased amount of fat in the diet, typical of the high-fat Western diet. In countries where fat intake is low, such as rural China, girls reach puberty between ages 15 and 19.

Late Menopause

Late menopause is defined as occurring after age 55. The increased risk is associated with the longer time a woman ovulates and thus has estrogen circulating through her body. It is common for women who begin to menstruate early to have a late menopause; thus, they may have up to 10 additional years of high estrogen levels. Compared with women who have a late menopause, those who go through the change before age 45 have half the risk of breast cancer.

Pregnancy and Breast-Feeding

Because pregnancy and breast-feeding reduce the number of menstrual cycles you go through and therefore the amount of estrogen in the body, both have an effect on your risk of breast cancer. Here's an overview of what researchers have found:

- Women who give birth when they are younger than 30 have a lower risk of breast cancer than do women who conceive after age 30 or who never give birth.

- Being pregnant increases a woman's risk of breast cancer for several years after she gives birth, especially among women who conceive after age 30.

- Having breast-fed reduces a woman's risk of breast cancer while she is premenopausal but offers no protection when she is postmenopausal.

- Generally, the younger you are when you breast-feed and the longer you do it, the greater the protection.

Estrogen and Hormone Replacement Therapy

Many doctors recommend estrogen or hormone replacement therapy for women as they go through menopause because it can reduce the risk of osteoporosis and heart disease. However, there is strong evidence that long-term and perhaps even short-term use of these hormone therapies place women at a greatly increased risk of breast cancer. This topic, which is controversial, is discussed in Chapter 6. Here it is simply noted that estrogen and hormone replacement therapy are significant risk factors for breast cancer, and that there are safe, natural alternatives for women who want to prevent osteoporosis and heart disease, as well as menopausal symptoms, including diet (see Chapter 4) and supplements (see Chapter 5).

Obesity and Weight Gain

Several studies show that being overweight as an adult is a risk factor for breast cancer. According to a Harvard School of Public Health study, in which more than 95,000 women were evaluated, women who gain 22 to 44 pounds after age 18 have a 60% increased risk of breast cancer. Most studies find the risk is greatest for postmenopausal women.

The factor that links obesity and breast cancer is estrogen. Estrogen is produced by abdominal fat cells, which transform other hormones, like testosterone, into estrogen. Women who carry a lot of weight around their abdomen have higher levels of estrogen circulating through their body. This added weight is not a problem among premenopausal women, because they have higher levels of specific proteins that reduce the amount of free estrogen in the body. However, obesity is a risk factor for other diseases, including diabetes, heart disease, and stroke, and so younger women who are overweight are not protected against health problems. The other clear danger is that in most cases overweight younger women remain overweight their entire life and therefore they carry the risk with them.

Breast Implants

Another area of controversy in breast cancer is the risk associated with implants. In 1987, the Food and Drug Administration (FDA) uncovered an unpublished report by Dow Corning in which the implant manufacturer stated that their silicone gel implants caused an increase in the incidence of malignant tumors in rats. The FDA and Corning then buried the information, and even when it was resurrected in 1990 by the Ralph Nader Health Research Group, Dow claimed that their findings didn't have any relevance to humans.

Few studies of the negative effects of silicone gel implants have been released, and some experts believe this is because the implant industry and the FDA continue to ignore, suppress, or trivialize the dangers. Over the years, a few industry whistle-blowers wrote private memos about the cancer-causing properties of the implants. Some of these memos and implant industry studies were revealed in 1992 in major publications, such as the *New York Times* and *Medical Tribune*, and then again in 1995 in the *International Journal of Occupational Medicine and Toxicology*, as well as in information received through the Freedom of Information Act and confidential sources.

The exact risk of breast cancer from silicone gel implants is unclear. If you have breast implants, detection of breast cancer using regular mammography is unreliable. However, magnetic resonance imaging (MRI) can penetrate the silicone. Some experts recommend removal of the implants to reduce the risk of cancer as well as leakage of the implant (which has occurred in more than 3000 women) or the possibility of developing an autoimmune disease. A 1993 study reports that up to 35% of women with silicone gel implants develop autoantibodies, substances that can cause rheumatoid arthritis, scleroderma, and systemic lupus erythematosus.

Another possible cancer risk related to breast implants is associated with the polyurethane foam that is used to cover some silicone gel implants. This foam, which is used as an industrial insulation material, is made from the carcinogen 2,4-toluene diisocyanate and is more carcinogenic than the gel.

In the late 1990s, several studies were published that essentially exonerated silicone gel implants (see Chapter 12). By then, however, saline-filled implants had taken their place, although the shell is made of silicone. Thus far, it is uncertain whether saline implants pose a cancer risk.

Other Risk Factors

The risk factors mentioned above play a role in whether a woman will get breast cancer. However, the fact is that these factors are not involved in about 70% of breast cancer cases. As mentioned earlier, according to the American Cancer Research Institute, environmental and lifestyle factors are responsible for about 70% of cancers. Many of those environmental and lifestyle causes are discussed in detail in Chapter 9.

Diagnosis Cancer: Now What?

If your biopsy results indicate malignancy, call in a general surgeon if you have not already. This specialist should provide you with a full explanation of all your options and a complete report on how each procedure is performed, the side effects, and what to expect. To help you choose a doctor, refer to "How to Select a Breast Specialist" on the following page.

How to Select a Breast Specialist

- Ask for referrals from your general practitioner, family and friends, the American Cancer Society, and other cancer organizations. If there is a teaching hospital or medical school–affiliated hospital in your area, ask them for recommendations. Teaching hospitals and medical schools have access to the latest developments and technology.

- Check out the credentials and qualifications of your candidates. You want a physician who is board certified, which means she or he has completed the necessary training and practice in her or his specialty. *The Directory of Medical Specialists*, available in the reference section of most libraries, provides a wealth of information on physicians. You can also contact the American Board of Medical Specialists (www.certifieddoctor.com).

- Select a physician who has experience in treating breast cancer patients. Ask if the doctor works as part of a breast cancer team. A team approach is a common one and offers you well-rounded and comprehensive treatment.

- Meet with potential physician(s) and note manner, personality, and sensitivity. Is he or she easy to talk to? Does he or she answer your questions (see below) and display a sincere interest in your questions and ideas? Are explanations understandable? Does he or she take enough time or does he or she seem impatient when you ask questions?

If you get a diagnosis of breast cancer, you need time to think and plan before you act. Surround yourself with support from family, friends, and medical experts. Part of that support includes getting a second opinion and a surgeon you trust, who respects your opinions, and who values your questions. No question is stupid or trivial. Some questions you could ask include:

- Where will the procedure be done, and does it require local or general anesthesia?
- What is the least invasive procedure available for my situation?
- How long will I be in the hospital?
- How will the surgery affect my mobility?
- How much scarring can I expect after the procedure?
- Can I have breast reconstruction if I need it?
- What are the chances that the cancer will spread?
- Will I need radiation, chemotherapy, or hormone therapy?
- What are the side effects of treatment?
- Which complementary treatments can I use?

You will be establishing a long-term relationship with a breast management team that includes your surgeon, your primary care physician, a medical oncologist, and possibly a radiation oncologist, an oncology nurse, a plastic surgeon, and a practitioner of complementary medicine (see "Complementary Medicine for Breast Cancer," later in this chapter). Ask questions. Write them down so that you won't forget them. Take notes when you get answers. Working together as a team can help make the experience easier for you and you can go about the business of healing that much better.

Treatment: Surgery and Radiation

Surgery and radiation are the primary methods women pursue to treat breast cancer, yet they are not the only methods available. There are literally dozens of cancer treatments—several have some sound scientific basis, but many do not. Some in the former category are discussed in Chapters 4, 5, and 7, and at the end of this chapter. They are primarily complementary therapies, designed to enhance the benefits of and reduce the need for conventional treatment, alleviate the side effects associated with it, and improve overall quality of life. Complementary treatments should not be used in place of conventional therapy without the approval of your medical doctor.

Surgery and Radiation

The primary conventional treatment for breast cancer is surgery, but the extent of that surgery has changed dramatically over the years. At one time, removal of one or both breasts (mastectomy) was the norm, but this approach has been replaced in most cases by breast-conserving and skin-sparing surgeries along with radiation treatment for most women with stage I or II cancer. Studies comparing these less radical surgeries with mastectomy show that they are equally effective. A look at different surgical procedures follows, along with an explanation of the radiation treatment that may accompany them.

LUMPECTOMY Lumpectomy is a type of breast-conserving surgery in which the surgeon removes only the cancerous mass and some of the normal breast tissue that surrounds it. The surgeon also usually removes some of the axillary lymph nodes, a procedure called axillary node dissection, which is discussed below.

After a lumpectomy, radiation treatment of the entire breast is initiated to kill any cancer cells that may still remain. Treatment consists of a daily dose of radiation, 5 days a week, for 5 to 6 weeks. At the end of this cycle, a single boost of radiation is given to the site where the tumor was removed.

The radiation used to treat lumpectomy typically does not cause major side effects, such as hair loss, fatigue, or nausea. You may experience temporary reddening of the breast skin after several weeks of receiving radiation, and the reddening may linger for several weeks after treatment is completed. About 25% of women who have had axillary node dissection experience edema (swelling) of the breast, accompanied by slight thickening of the skin.

Not every woman who has a lumpectomy needs radiation. If the tumor is noninvasive and the lymph nodes are not involved, radiation may not be necessary.

REGIONAL LYMPH NODE DISSECTION   If the cancer has spread to the lymph nodes, there are four options: surgical removal (which may be followed by radiation), chemotherapy, hormone treatment, or radiation treatment. The axillary nodes are the ones most often involved, with occasional cases affecting the internal mammary or supraclavicular (collarbone area) lymph nodes. The number of nodes affected indicates the risk that there will be microscopic spread of the cancer to other parts of the body. The greater number of nodes involved, the higher the risk.

If the nodes are not enlarged, radiation can be used to treat them. Radiation is also an option when physicians believe no additional useful information can be gathered by examining the nodes, or when there is a possibility the cancer may spread to the internal mammary or supraclavicular nodes.

Frequently, surgeons perform axillary node dissection, which is removal of the lymph nodes that lie below the axillary vein and those between the major chest wall muscles and the major back muscle. This surgery can be done along with standard or skin-sparing mastectomy, breast reconstruction, or breast-conserving procedures. Recent studies suggest that some women may benefit from chemotherapy rather than dissection.

SENTINEL NODE BIOPSY   Sentinel node biopsy is a new procedure in which only the first (sentinel) or a few additional axillary nodes are removed through a small incision instead of an entire node dissection. This less invasive procedure greatly reduces postoperative discomfort and recovery time. Not every woman is a candidate, so you need to discuss this option with your physician.

SAYING NO TO LUMPECTOMY AND RADIATION   In some cases, breast-conserving surgery and radiation are not recommended. If you are pregnant, radiation can cause birth defects and increase the chance that your child will develop cancer or leukemia. Lumpectomy and node dissection can be performed during pregnancy, but radiation needs to wait until after the infant is delivered. Other reasons to avoid lumpectomy and radiation include:

- Previous radiation therapy to the involved breast. Women who were treated with radiation for a prior condition, such as Hodgkin's disease, should not undergo lumpectomy or radiation. Added radiation to the breast can cause severe ulceration or scarring.

- The presence of lupus or scleroderma. Women with these diseases can experience severe scarring of the breast if they undergo lumpectomy and radiation.

- Two separate cancers in the same breast. Lumpectomy and radiation may still be an option if you meet certain criteria. Therefore, the options should be discussed with your surgeon.

- The mammogram shows extensive malignant microcalcifications throughout the breast. Microcalcifications are minute flecks of calcium that signify small amounts of cancer. If they are distributed widely throughout the breast, mastectomy is the more logical choice.

Some women, after learning about the surgical and radiation options, elect to have a mastectomy even when lumpectomy and radiation are indicated. An overwhelming fear that the cancer will return, lack of a strong desire to preserve the breast, a physical inability to undergo radiation (for example, severe arthritis that makes it impossible to lie flat for radiation treatments), or an intense fear of radiation may make mastectomy a better choice for some women.

MASTECTOMY   Removal of the entire breast and often part of the adjacent chest muscle is no longer considered to be the only safe treatment for breast cancer. In about 30% of women with breast cancer it is the only sensible choice, because of the severity of the disease. The purpose of mastectomy is to remove all of the cancerous tissue to minimize the possibility of local recurrence and to prevent spread to other parts of the body. Mastectomy can be radical, modified radical, or simple.

Radical mastectomy involves removal of the entire breast plus the underlying chest wall muscles and the axillary lymph nodes. It is rarely used today, but at one time it was the primary way to deal with breast cancer.

Modified radical mastectomy has largely replaced the radical procedure and is just as effective. This modified version preserves the largest chest wall muscle, the pectoralis major, which helps support the breasts. Women who want to have breast reconstruction can elect to have it done during the same operation or at a later time.

Total or simple mastectomy involves removal of the breast but not the lymph nodes. If there is no tumor involvement of the skin, the woman may elect to have skin-sparing mastectomy performed. This procedure results in a better cosmetic effect than a regular simple mastectomy.

RADIATION AFTER MASTECTOMY   Evidence regarding the benefits of radiation treatment after mastectomy is inconclusive, and there's no strong proof that this combination improves the chances of cure. Many physicians recommend radiation for women who are at high risk of recurrence, such as those who had large tumors, enlarged axillary lymph nodes, or many lymph nodes with metastases.

Chemotherapy

Chemotherapy is the use of drugs to damage or kill cancer cells throughout the body. It is typically used after breast surgery and can be combined with radiation or hormonal therapy. Infrequently, chemotherapy is started before surgery, especially in cases of advanced cancer or when a large tumor rules out breast-conserving surgery. Chemotherapy is usually started 4 to 6 weeks after surgery and continues for about 4 to

8 months. Most of the drugs must be given intravenously, although there are a few oral forms.

A chemotherapy regimen is highly individual, chosen to meet a patient's unique needs. Generally, chemotherapy drugs hinder or block the reproduction and growth of malignant cells. Because cancer cells tend to grow faster than normal cells, they absorb the drug more readily and hopefully die before too much damage is done to surrounding healthy cells. The most common and less common chemotherapy drugs are listed below, along with some of the combination therapies in which two or more drugs are administered.

Chemotherapy Drugs for Breast Cancer

Commonly Used Drugs:

- Cyclophosphamide (Cytoxan) [C]. The most frequently administered alkylating agent, a class that also includes melphalan, thiotepa, cisplatin, and carboplatin. Cyclophosphamide suppresses bone marrow and can cause hair loss, bladder toxicity, and premature menopause.

- Doxorubicin (Adriamycin) [A]. A very powerful drug used to treat recurrent and metastatic cancer. It causes hair loss, bone marrow suppression, and mouth sores. Adriamycin can damage the heart muscle, but administration of a compound called ICRF-187 offers protection. A natural protectant is coenzyme Q10 (see Chapter 5).

- 5-Fluorouracil (5-FU) [F]. In a class that also includes methotrexate. Side effects are mouth sores, nerve damage, and diarrhea. It also has been linked with fertility problems in women.

- Methotrexate [M]. An antimetabolite. Side effects include mouth sores and, rarely, fibrosis of the lungs. It can also damage the kidneys, which can be prevented or significantly reduced by taking the folic acid derivative leucovorin and other supplements (see Chapter 5).

- Prednisone [P]. A corticosteroid used in combination therapy to enhance the cancer-killing powers of other drugs.
- Vincristine (Oncovin) [V]. A derivative of the periwinkle plant. It can cause severe skin damage if it leaks from the IV at the injection site. Hair loss is common, and nerve damage can occur, especially in individuals who have pre-existing neuropathy.

Common Drug Combinations:

CMF (Cytoxan + methotrexate + 5-FU)

CAF (Cytoxan + Adriamycin + 5-FU)

AC (Adriamycin + Cytoxan)

CMFP (CMF + prednisone)

CAFMV (CAF + methotrexate + vincristine)

Less-Commonly Used Drugs:

Docetaxel (Taxotere)

Mitomycin-C

Mitoxantrone (Novantrone)

Paclitaxel (Taxol)

Thiotepa (Thioplex)

Vinorelbine (Navelbine)

Perhaps the most dreaded aspects of chemotherapy are the side effects, which often include hair loss, nausea, vomiting, and low blood counts. These problems occur because the cells in the scalp and stomach also grow quickly, so they are killed by the chemotherapy as well. Not every drug causes all of these side effects, and not every woman experiences them. Chemotherapy also damages bone marrow cells, which can compromise the immune system and an individual's survival. Other side effects include mouth sores, tingling in the toes and fingers, disruption of the menstrual cycle, and fatigue. More severe complications include scarring of the heart muscle, bladder irritation, lung complications, skin ulcers, and kidney problems. Physicians often prescribe other medications to offset the more serious side effects, including growth factors to help maintain white blood cell counts and antinausea drugs. Natural remedies can reduce the severity of side effects and boost the immune system (see Chapter 5).

Hormonal Therapy

Hormonal therapy allows women to control breast cancer by modifying the balance of hormone levels in their body, essentially blocking the supply of estrogen that breast cancer cells need to grow. The hormone receptor test discussed previously is used to select which patients may benefit from hormone therapy. About half of all patients who have positive estrogen receptors will benefit from hormonal treatment, compared with less than 10% of those with negative receptors.

Antiestrogen Therapy

One of the best-known hormonal drugs is tamoxifen (Nolvadex), an antiestrogen therapy used by women who have positive estrogen or progesterone receptors. Tamoxifen attaches itself to estrogen receptors in the breast and prevents natural estrogen from latching on and promoting cancer growth. Tamoxifen, along with the other antiestrogen drug toremifene (Fareston), is used in both pre- and postmenopausal women who are at risk of recurrence of breast cancer after surgery and who have receptor-positive tumors. The use of tamoxifen for 5 years in such women reportedly reduces the risk of recurrent cancer by 50%. This benefit is over and above any reduction gained from chemotherapy.

Commonly Used Hormonal Therapy Drugs
Antiestrogens

    Tamoxifen (Nolvadex)
    Toremifene (Fareston)

Progestational Hormones

Megestrol acetate (Megace)

Aromatase Inhibitors

Anastrozole (Arimidex)

Letrozole (Femara)

Antiestrogens cause few side effects (hot flashes, vaginal dryness), but do carry a small risk of uterine cancer. Uncommon adverse reactions include weight gain, blood clots, vaginal bleeding, nausea, rash, muscle cramps, and low blood count. When antiestrogens are given along with chemotherapy, there is an increased risk of blood clots. An advantage of antiestrogens is that they strengthen bone in postmenopausal women and reduce serum cholesterol levels.

The long-term effects of tamoxifen are being investigated in a large (16,000 pre- and postmenopausal women) study. The results of the NCI/NSABP (National Cancer Institute/ National Surgical Adjuvant Breast Project) Breast Cancer Prevention Trial will not be available until 2002 or 2003. Physicians hope the findings will settle the question of whether tamoxifen is safe to use in premenopausal women, as well as identify any long-term consequences of its use.

Other Hormonal Therapies

Progestational hormones, such as megestrol acetate (Megace) or medroxyprogesterone acetate (Provera) are prescribed for some women. Although these drugs have fewer side effects than antiestrogens, they cause an increase in appetite, which usually leads to weight gain. Fluid retention is also common.

A new class of drugs, called aromatase inhibitors, is for advanced breast cancer in postmenopausal women who do not respond to tamoxifen. Currently there are two available, anastrozole (Arimidex) and letrozole (Femara). Aromatase inhibitors block the production of aromatase, which then blocks production of estrogen. Side effects include enlarged breasts, hair loss, blood clots in the lungs, and phlebitis of veins. Because these drugs block estrogen production, women lose estrogen's bone-building and cardiovascular benefits.

Complementary Medicine for Breast Cancer

At the Eleventh International Congress on Women's Health Issues held in San Francisco in January 2000, University of California, San Francisco, researchers announced the results of a 5-year study that examined the use of alternative therapies among white, Latino, and Asian women with breast cancer. They found that more than 70% of breast cancer patients use some form of complementary therapy, including acupuncture, herbs, nutritional supplements, or prayer, but only one-third of the women disclose this information to their physicians. Reasons for not telling their medical doctors about the alternative treatment include having the impression their physician is not interested, is unwilling or unable to provide relevant information, or would disapprove. Although most of the women did not expect their medical doctors to endorse the complementary practices, they did want the physicians to respect their choice, and to be open-minded and willing to listen.

In another study, 379 women with breast cancer from four ethnic groups—white, black, Latino, and Asian—were asked about their use of conventional and alternative cancer treatments. The findings revealed that about 50% of the women used at least one alternative therapy, and about 33% used two. Black women used spiritual healing (36%), Chinese women used herbal remedies (22%), and Latinos used both dietary therapies (30%) and spiritual healing (26%). White women used dietary (35%) and physical therapies (massage, acupuncture, and others; 21%). More than 90% of the women said the therapies were helpful.

These two studies illustrate several important points. One is that although women are using conventional therapies, complementary approaches are clearly important to them. Another is that patients report that complementary cancer therapies can be instrumental in the healing process.

But perhaps the most important point is that at least half of women are not telling their medical doctors about their alternative treatments. Some complementary practices are powerful and can significantly impact conventional treatments. (Explore complementary approaches in Chapters 4, 5, and 7.) Patients need to discuss their self-chosen therapies with their physician, and physicians must educate themselves and listen. If you are looking for a physician to manage your breast cancer and you want to explore nontraditional treatments, select a doctor who respects your choices and will work with you. Although all patient–doctor relationships are important, the one between you as a woman with breast cancer and your physician should be especially based on trust and respect. It just may be the relationship that saves your life.

Nothing about breast cancer is simple. It can be caused by different factors, treated various ways, and spread to many different parts of the body. Everywhere you turn, there is controversy about breast cancer, whether it be about the role of saturated fat, questions about whether mammography is safe or how often women should get routine mammograms, or the sensitive issue of testing for breast cancer genes. With so much debate surrounding it, breast cancer is always in the news if not in laboratories and clinical trials around the world. And there is good news in this revolving controversy, because it fosters more research and hopefully more answers.

But not every problem a woman has with her breasts involves cancer. More often than not, the lumps, bumps, and pain are associated with benign conditions. In the next chapter, you will learn about these noncancerous breast problems.

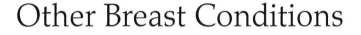

Other Breast Conditions

Millions of women have been sent home from the doctor with a diagnosis of fibrocystic breast disease, unsure about what this means. The word *disease* sounds foreboding. Even though many of these women probably were also told not to worry about their "disease," the psychological damage had been done.

Fibrocystic breast disease is just a convenient, albeit inaccurate, term that many doctors still use to describe the pain and any one of the various types of benign lumps or cysts that affect approximately 50% of women. In 1985, the American Cancer Society's National Task Force on Breast Cancer Control announced that "fibrocystic breast disease" was an unacceptable term. With the help of the College of American Pathologists, they decided on "benign breast changes" and divided the condition into three groups: breast changes with no increased risk for breast cancer, those with a slightly increased risk, and those with a moderately increased risk.

This method of grouping benign breast changes is not the only approach, however. Dr. Susan Love, author of *Dr. Susan Love's Breast Book* and *Dr. Susan Love's Hormone Book: Making Informed Choices About Menopause*, and a well-known spokesperson on women's health issues, developed a more precise way to explain benign breast changes. Her categories include:

- Normal physical changes, including swelling, lumps, cysts, and mild tenderness; commonly referred to as cyclic fibrocystic changes
- Severe breast pain (mastalgia)
- Inflammation and infections
- Nipple problems (including discharge and cracking)
- Abnormal amount of lumpiness
- Dominant benign lumps

This chapter explores the different benign breast conditions that can affect women of all ages. Although the breast problems discussed here are often painful and uncomfortable, and can occasionally make it difficult to detect breast tumors, they are not life-threatening. Knowledge is your best weapon against them. Here you will come to better understand your breast condition so that you will be better prepared to deal with it, using the suggestions provided with each explanation.

College of American Pathologists

Relative Risk of Breast Cancer
According to Benign Change

RELATIVE RISK   An estimate of the probability that a woman with a benign breast condition will develop breast cancer, as compared with a woman who has no known significant breast abnormality.

NO INCREASED RISK   Conditions that have no signs of hyperplasia (excessive cell growth): apocrine metaplasia, duct ectasa, fibroadenoma, fibrocystic changes, mild hyperplasia, mastitis.

SLIGHTLY INCREASED RISK (1.5 TO 2 TIMES)   Moderate or severe hyperplasia, papilloma, sclerosing adenosis.

MODERATELY INCREASED RISK (5 TIMES)   Atypical hyperplasia of the ductal or lobular type.

The Anatomy of Change

The breast is composed of two types of tissues: glandular and stromal (supporting). The glandular tissue includes the lobules, which produce milk; and the ducts, which are passageways that carry milk to the nipples. Each breast is divided into 15 to 20 sections, called lobes, which are cushioned by fat cells. Each lobe consists of several lobules, and each lobule has several tiny sacs called acini (or alveoli). These sacs extract needed substances from surrounding blood vessels to produce milk.

The stromal tissue includes fibrous connective tissues, which are the ligaments that support the breast (called Cooper's ligaments) and fatty tissue. Any of the glandular or stromal tissues can react to fluctuations in hormone levels and hormonal messages that may result in either cancerous or benign breast conditions. (Breast cancer is discussed in Chapter 10.) Benign breast problems are discussed below.

Cyclic Fibrocystic Change

According to the American Cancer Society, about 50% of women experience cyclic fibrocystic change sometime during their life. Some women say they can set their calendars by it. The "it" is the monthly occurrence of breast tenderness, pain, and swelling that many women of childbearing age experience before their menstrual cycle. This condition is referred to by various names: breast pain, cyclic fibrocystic changes, and cyclic breast changes are just a few of them. Call it what you like, but it is not a disease, nor is it dangerous.

Why Your Breasts Hurt

Throughout the menstrual cycle, and especially during the 2 weeks before the period starts, it is normal for the glandular tissue in the breasts to feel lumpy (nodular). Pain and tenderness often occur as well. These symptoms are the result of extra blood and other body fluids that accumulate in the breast tissue during this part of the menstrual cycle. Some women have more lumps, pain, or tenderness than others, depending on how sensitive their breast tissue is to hormonal changes, their age (women in their 30s often have more discomfort than younger women), and their hormone balance. After menopause, these symptoms stop, unless you take hormone therapy. Severe breast pain is called mastalgia and does not appear to be related to menstrual cycle changes in most cases (see below).

All of this pain and tenderness makes it difficult if not impossible to do a thorough breast examination. That's one reason why women are encouraged to do their breast self-exams after their menstrual cycle, when the pain and tenderness are gone. Another reason is that during the 2 weeks before your period your breasts are especially lumpy, which makes it hard to detect any abnormalities.

Scientists have not found any significant relationship between fibrocystic change and breast cancer, and the condition rarely requires surgical treatment. Researchers know that hormones are involved in this cycle of breast pain, but they don't know exactly how or why they cause symptoms. They can't blame the high or low levels of any one particular hormone, because women with both high and low hormone levels experience symptoms. One popular theory is that the hormone receptors in the breast vary in their sensitivity, which ultimately depends on the level of essential fatty acids in the body.

Treatment

Until experts can more clearly identify the cause of cyclic fibrocystic changes, there will continue to be many different treatments offered. Several natural approaches that have proven effective in dealing with the pain and discomfort are elimination of caffeine (see Chapter 9), eating a low-fat diet (Chapter 4), and maintaining a reasonable body weight. One study found that a low-fat (15% fat) diet significantly reduced breast tenderness, swelling, and nodularity in 60% of women compared with only 20% in a control group. Foods that contain hormones, such as beef, pork, chicken, and dairy products, also should be avoided. Foods that can help relieve symptoms include citrus, beets, carrots, celery, artichokes, spinach, and cucumbers.

Supplements that have proven helpful include vitamins A, B_6, C, and E, and evening primrose oil. If fluid retention is causing the pain, herbal diuretics can be helpful (see Chapter 5). See below for an overview of treatment options for fibrocystic breast changes.

TREATMENTS FOR FIBROCYSTIC BREAST CHANGES

- Wear an extra-support bra.
- Eliminate caffeine (see Chapter 9).
- Take pain relievers, such as ibuprofen or aspirin.
- Apply warm compresses to the breasts (see Chapter 5 for formulations).
- Reduce your salt intake (helps reduce swelling).
- Take oral contraceptives (this is controversial; nondrug approaches should always be tried before resorting to drugs).

- Take diuretics (herbal preferred; see Chapter 5).
- Take nutritional supplements (see Chapter 5).
- Take bromocriptine or danazol (prescription drugs for severe cases only. Both drugs can cause serious side effects, including nausea, dizziness, and fertility problems associated with bromocriptine; and weight gain, amenorrhea, and growth of facial hair with danazol.).
- Have the growth drained using fine-needle aspiration.
- Have breast lumps surgically removed (should be the last resort).

Mastalgia (Severe Breast Pain)

Approximately 8 to 10% of premenopausal women experience moderate to severe breast pain, or mastalgia, every month. For many of these women, the pain recurs every month for years, often until they reach menopause.

Mastalgia is a recognized symptom of premenstrual syndrome (PMS), even though not every woman who has PMS experiences severe breast pain. A recent study conducted at the Uniformed Services University of the Health Sciences in Bethesda, Maryland, revealed that most women with mastalgia do not have PMS. Indeed, 82% of the women in the study who had cyclical mastalgia did not have PMS symptoms. Therefore, even though cyclical mastalgia seems to be associated with the menstrual cycle, the investigators report that it is "not simply premenstrual syndrome, and merits further investigation as a recurrent pain disorder."

Women are encouraged to try natural approaches to relieve the pain of mastalgia. Chapter 5 offers several options.

Breast Cysts

A cyst is a type of lump that is filled with fluid. It can be microscopic (2 millimeters or smaller, called microcysts) or as big as a golf ball (3 millimeters or larger, called macrocysts). Cysts appear in women between the ages of 16 and 50 and are often tender or painful. The most common spot for cysts is the upper outer portion of the breast, where they can be surrounded by milk ducts, fatty tissue, and milk glands. It is not uncommon for women in their late 30s and 40s to regularly develop cysts, because their hormones are undergoing changes as they prepare for menopause. There is some evidence that a lack of iodine, which can cause symptoms of an underactive thyroid gland, can also cause breast cysts. Wearing a bra day and night, especially if it has underwires, may make you susceptible to breast cysts.

Cysts usually feel soft and smooth, or, if they are deep in the breast, they may feel hard. If the lump does not disappear within a menstrual cycle, it should be drained by your physician to determine if the lump is benign. This procedure is known as a fine-needle aspiration, and it is usually done in the doctor's office (see Chapter 10).

Preventing and Treating Cysts

Eating a diet that's rich in vegetables, fruits, and whole grains and that avoids meat and dairy products is helpful. Women who eat a plant-based diet eliminate two to three times more detoxified estrogens than women who eat meat, and thus reduce their risk of cyst formation. Products containing caffeine should be avoided.

Supplements shown to help improve the symptoms of breast cysts include vitamin E, kelp, beta-carotene, vitamin C, chaste tree, evening primrose oil, and B vitamins. See Chapter 5 for information on these natural remedies.

Drug treatment for breast cysts includes the only drug approved by the FDA for this purpose. Danazol (Danocrine) is derived from testosterone and works to block the release of two hormones, FSH (follicle-stimulating hormone) and LH (luteinizing hormone). The result is that estrogen production is blocked. Side effects include weight gain, acne, bloating, and irregular bleeding.

Cysts and Breast Cancer

The link between breast cysts and breast cancer is cloudy. Some studies suggest that women with macrocysts have a 2- to 4-fold increased risk of breast cancer, but other studies show little or no increased risk. One study analyzed the fluid of the cysts from more than 1000 women and found a 5-fold increased risk of breast cancer in those who had a high potassium:sodium ratio compared with a low ratio. This is an interesting theory, but its value has yet to be determined.

If after one or more aspirations the cyst recurs in the same location, your doctor may want to do a biopsy. Even if it is benign, such recurrence is suspicious and may warrant removing the growth to prevent possible cancer growth.

Benign Breast Lumps

Fibroadenomas

Young women in their teens and 20s are the most likely candidates for this type of benign breast tumor. When analyzed according to racial group, the American Cancer Society reports that black women develop these tumors more than any other ethnic or racial group. Fibroadenomas are firm, rounded, rubbery tumors that are nearly always benign and are unrelated to breast cancer. They are composed of structural (fibro) and glandular (adenoma) tissue and typically move around easily when felt. Usually, however, they are too small to be palpated. Some women have only one tumor whereas others develop several.

Women with fibroadenomas who become pregnant or who are breast-feeding may notice that the tumors enlarge during those times. This is normal and does not indicate that they are malignant. Fine-needle aspiration or core-needle biopsy can be used to make a definitive diagnosis of these tumors. Because fibroadenomas often stop growing or shrink without any treatment, physicians typically adopt a wait-and-see approach. If the tumors continue to grow or do not shrink, most surgeons recommend removing them.

Intraductal Papilloma

Intraductal papillomas are benign, wart-like tumors that grow into the breast ducts near the nipple. They can be solitary, which is common among women who are approaching menopause, or multiple. Papillomas are very sensitive to touch, and any slight bump near the nipple can cause the papilloma to bleed or to leak a sticky discharge from the nipple. In rare cases, the discharge becomes bothersome, in which case the damaged duct can be surgically removed. Physicians usually use a procedure called duct excision to diagnose these growths.

Multiple papillomas are common among younger women and usually occur in both breasts. These papillomas are more often associated with a lump than with nipple discharge. Generally, any woman who has multiple intraductal papillomas or any papilloma that is associated with a lump should have the growth(s) removed.

Fat Necrosis

Fat necrosis is a painless, round, firm lump that results from an injury to the breast or from disintegrating fatty tissue. It is common among women who are obese and who have very large breasts. The skin surrounding the lumps may be red or bruised. Most physicians recommend that fat necrosis be removed and a biopsy performed, because these lumps are easily mistaken for cancer.

According to the American Cancer Society, some women respond differently to a breast injury. Instead of scar tissue forming at the injured site, the fat cells die and release their contents, which then form an oil cyst. Oil cysts can be diagnosed using fine-needle aspiration, which can also be used to drain them.

Sclerosing Adenosis

The appearance of excessive tissue growth in the breast's lobules is a benign condition known as sclerosing adenosis. The condition is characterized by minute, usually microscopic lumps that can be detected on mammography as calcifications, small deposits of calcium in the tissues. Calcifications are common in women older than 50 and are seen occasionally in younger women. More than 80% of them are benign.

Widely scattered calcifications in one or both breasts typically do not cause any concern, but a cluster in one breast may suggest intraductal cancer. Because a mammogram cannot distinguish between benign and malignant calcifications, a biopsy is necessary. If you are younger than 35, chances are very good that the deposits are benign, but it is still important to get a definite diagnosis as quickly as possible (within 4 to 6 weeks) because cancer in younger women generally grows faster than it does in older women. (See Chapter 10 for information on a biopsy.)

Duct Ectasia

Also known as mammary duct ectasia, this disease affects women who are approaching menopause. This often painful condition occurs when the ducts beneath the nipple become clogged and inflamed. The result is a thick, sticky, gray-green discharge from the nipples. The nipple and the area surrounding it may be tender and red. Many cases of duct ectasia respond well to hot compresses (see herbal treatments in Chapter 5 under "Nipple Pain"). Physicians usually prescribe antibiotics and, in severe cases, may recommend surgical removal of the duct.

Mastitis

Mastitis is a bacterial infection of the breast ducts and nipple. It is most often seen in women who are breast-feeding, but it does occur in women who are not. Typical characteristics of mastitis include cracking of the skin around the nipple, swelling, and red, painful breasts that are warm to the touch. Mastitis occurs when bacteria, such as *Staphylococcus aureus* or *Streptococcus*, enter the breast duct through the skin cracks. Fever occurs in some women.

Many physicians prescribe an antibiotic, but other, natural options are available, including homeopathic remedies and application of hot compresses to relieve the pain (see Chapter 5). If an abscess containing pus forms, it needs to be drained.

If your physician tells you that you have fibrocystic breast changes, ask for a detailed explanation. You are most likely experiencing symptoms caused by hormonal fluctuations or a benign breast change. An inaccurate diagnosis of fibrocystic breast disease on an insurance form can result in your insurance carrier refusing to cover your medical costs, as well as cause you additional coverage problems down the road.

Most benign breast problems can be resolved using homemade and nondrug treatments: herbs, massage, compresses, and homeopathic remedies. See Chapter 5 for suggestions.

✿

CHAPTER TWELVE

All about Surgery: Cosmetic and Reconstructive

When a woman makes an appointment with a surgeon for cosmetic breast changes, she does so for various reasons. One may be purely cosmetic: she wants her breasts to be bigger, smaller, higher, or more symmetrical. In some cases, especially for breast reduction, there may be medical reasons as well. Very large breasts can contribute to or cause back, neck, and shoulder pain, which breast reduction can resolve. Another reason is for breast reconstruction following surgery for breast cancer. Statistics show that whereas only about 20% of women who had a mastectomy in the 1980s elected to have breast reconstruction, more than 80% are choosing that option today.

This chapter discusses both cosmetic and reconstructive breast changes. You will learn what questions to ask yourself and your surgeon when you are contemplating cosmetic breast surgery. You will read about how the procedures are done, their safety factor, and what outcome to expect. If you choose to forego surgery, we also discuss prostheses.

Cosmetic Breast Surgery

If you are contemplating changing the shape, size, or symmetry of your breasts, you first need to examine your motivations for doing so. Indeed, this should be one of the questions a plastic surgeon asks you when you are interviewing him or her as your possible choice of a surgeon. Then you need to do your homework, which includes choosing a surgeon and learning all you can about the procedure you have chosen.

Cosmetic breast surgery can be a positive, self-esteem-building experience or it can be a nightmare. To help ensure you have a positive experience, consider these guidelines.

Guidelines When Contemplating Cosmetic Breast Surgery

- Examine your reasons for wanting the surgery. They may be medical (breast reduction because of back pain) or personal (you're unhappy with the way your breasts look). The critical point is that *you* must be the one who wants the surgery—not your husband, boyfriend, family, or friend. If your response to "Why do you want cosmetic breast surgery?" is "My husband says I'd be more attractive if I had bigger breasts" or "My boyfriend says my breasts sag too much," then you are doing it to please someone else, not yourself, and you are setting yourself up for possible emotional conflicts or feelings of resentment.

- Identify your expectations. If you think new breasts will dramatically change your life, you are probably being unrealistic. If you expect to feel better about yourself and your appearance, those are more realistic goals.

- Have a support system in place. Breast surgery is a major event, both physical and emotional, and it will be helpful to have a partner, family member, or close friend who supports your decision.

- Choose a surgeon carefully. He or she should be board certified and experienced in the type of surgery you desire.

Contact the American Society of Plastic and Reconstructive Surgeons for referrals (see Resources). Also get recommendations from reliable people.

- Familiarize yourself with the procedures. Look for books, articles, and information on the Internet and in libraries about cosmetic breast surgery. Take notes and bring them with you when you interview potential candidates.

- Interview several candidates. Don't make a decision after talking with only one surgeon. This is an elective procedure, so don't rush. Arrange to talk with at least three plastic surgeons before you make your decision.

- Ask questions of your candidates. Any physician who seems reluctant to answer your questions should be taken off your list immediately. Ask for before and after pictures from patients they have had. Ask for referrals to other women who have had the type of surgery you are planning.

- Understand the risks. The surgeon should explain the positive and negative aspects of the procedure you are considering, including possible complications, the amount of postoperative pain to expect, and limitations after surgery.

- Ask about cost. Insurance companies typically do not cover cosmetic breast surgery unless it can be proven that breast reduction is necessary for health reasons. Some insurance companies require that a certain percentage of tissue be removed in order for the surgery to qualify for coverage.

Regardless of which procedure you choose or who does it, you should get a mammogram before surgery. This gives physicians a reference point for later mammograms. A baseline mammogram is especially important for women who elect augmentation, because it allows for any cysts to be addressed before the implants are placed. Your doctor will advise you to stop taking aspirin, vitamin E, nonsteroidal anti-inflammatory drugs, and other medications at least 2 weeks before surgery to help prevent bleeding complications.

All breast surgeries result in scarring, especially breast reductions. To help minimize scars, your first line of defense should be massage. Consult with your doctor about when you can safely begin to massage the affected area. Once you have your doctor's permission, massage the area in a circular motion two or three times a day for up to 20 minutes each time. Use aloe, vitamin E, or a mixture of the two to promote healing.

Breast Augmentation

Ever since the Food and Drug Administration (FDA) called for a delay in the use of silicone gel implants in January 1992, saline implants have been used almost exclusively for breast augmentation and, to a lesser extent, breast reconstruction. (See Chapter 10 for information on silicone gel implants.) According to the American Society of Plastic and Reconstructive Surgeons, more than 132,000 breast augmentations were performed in 1998, and 97 percent of them were saline implants.

Compared with silicone gel, saline reportedly feels less natural. But if the implant should leak, saline is safely absorbed by the body, whereas silicone cannot be broken down or used by the body. For these reasons, silicone gel was named as the cause of autoimmune diseases such as rheumatoid arthritis, lupus, and scleroderma by women who sued Dow Corning for defective silicone gel implants. Several studies published in the late 1990s did not prove that silicone gel implants caused these problems. However, they now are used only in clinical trials.

Choosing an Implant

Once you have decided to go ahead with breast augmentation, you need to decide whether you want a textured or smooth implant. Compared with smooth implants, *textured implants* are less likely to cause the formation of a capsular contracture. This shell of scar tissue often forms around a breast implant as the body reacts to the presence of a foreign body. A capsular contracture can make the breast feel harder or firmer than desired, and in some cases it is painful, although it is not dangerous. Most women say the additional firmness is acceptable, but sometimes it is so uncomfortable that women have the excess scar tissue removed in a procedure called a capsulotomy.

Textured implants have several drawbacks, however. They can cause a "rippling" effect, which can be seen along the edges of the implant. There is also some evidence that small particles of the silicone shell that encases saline implants may shed and enter the surrounding tissue. Silicone shedding is a concern for those who believe it may cause autoimmune disease, but this relationship has not been proven.

Although the rate of capsular contracture among smooth implants is greater than among the textured forms, the smooth implants are less likely to cause rippling, and no shedding has been observed. Overall, however, textured implants are chosen by women 2 to 1 over the smooth ones, primarily because of the reduced risk of capsular contracture.

Inserting a Breast Implant

An implant can be placed in one of two general areas: between the breast gland and the underlying muscle (*subglandular*), or under the muscles on the chest wall (*submuscular*). Submuscular implants are performed more often and are less likely to cause rippling or capsular contracture.

Placement of the incision can be under the armpit, around the areola, or in the fold under the breast. An armpit incision is less likely to affect sensation of the nipple, and it is generally a good choice for women who have a poorly defined breastfold or a small areola.

Breast augmentation generally can be done on an outpatient basis and takes about 1½ to 3 hours to complete. Recovery takes 5 to 7 days, after which you can resume normal activities. Strenuous exercise should be avoided for 4 to 6 weeks.

Possible Postsurgical Complications

About 18% of women who receive saline implants experience severe capsular contracture. This complication can occur as soon as 2 weeks to as long as 15 years after surgery. If you have smooth implants inserted, one way to help prevent scar formation is to massage the breasts twice a day. Ask your physician to illustrate the technique for you.

In about 2% of women, nipple sensation is lost or greatly reduced after implant surgery because the sensory nerves have been stretched. Some women have reduced feeling in their breasts as well.

Breast Reduction

Breast reduction, mammaplasty, is usually sought by women who are extremely uncomfortable and self-conscious about the size of their breasts. In most cases, the weight and volume of their breasts cause back and neck pain, as well as skin problems under the breasts, and rarely, skeletal problems. The American Society of Plastic Reconstructive Surgeons reports that more than 70,000 breast reductions were done in 1998.

Breast reduction involves more than simply removing tissue, although deciding how much tissue can be removed is one of the main questions women ask. The answer depends largely on the diameter of the breast, which is something a surgeon cannot change. Before you undergo a breast reduction, there are several points you and your surgeon need to clarify to ensure you fully understand what to expect:

- Agree on a size. B cup is the most popular request. If your surgeon believes that goal is not possible in your case, you may want a second opinion. Remember, just because you want to be a specific size does not necessarily mean it is a feasible or safe choice for you. The natural contours of your breast may not allow an extensive reduction.

- Know the risks. Breast reduction can cause lost or diminished nipple sensation, an inability to breast-feed (in about

50% of cases), and extensive scarring. Loss of nipple sensation is assured if the nipple and areola need to be removed and grafted higher on the breast. This is usually necessary in women who have very large breasts.

- Choose a procedure. Along with the traditional inverted T method, other breast reduction approaches include liposuction, the vertical scar or LeJour method, and the donut or Benelli reduction approach.

Doing the Procedure

Breast-reduction surgery is done in the hospital, typically takes 2 to 4 hours, and usually requires a 2- to 3-day hospital stay. After surgery you will likely have a tube in each breast for several days to drain excess fluids. You will also need to wear a surgical bra over gauze, and once the gauze is removed, you will continue to wear the surgical bra for several weeks. Overall, it takes about 6 to 12 months after breast reduction for the breasts to "settle" into their new shape.

Breast Lifts

Most of the women who seek a breast lift, or mastopexy, are between the ages of 35 and 50 and have sagging breasts due to pregnancy, breast-feeding, or gravity. No surgery, however, can permanently delay the effects of gravity on the breasts, so you cannot expect a breast lift to last forever. If you plan to become pregnant, postpone a breast lift until after you have your last child. Some women choose to have a breast lift and reduction or augmentation surgery at the same time in order to get the look they want. Discuss this option with your surgeon.

Of the two main mastopexy techniques—traditional and small-scar—the traditional method is considered to be more effective for severely sagging breasts. It involves incisions that are similar to those made for breast reduction (the T approach). In fact, a breast lift is similar to breast reduction except that a lift removes more skin than it does gland.

Small-scar mastopexy is best suited for women with minimal sag and excess skin. The only cut made is around the areola, and the skin and tissue is removed through the single incision. Only a small amount of skin can be removed using this approach.

Breast lifts can be done on an outpatient basis, and surgery typically lasts 1½ to 3½ hours. If breast reduction or augmentation is done at the same time, the procedure will last 1 hour or longer. After surgery you will need to wear a gauze wrap with a surgical bra for a few days, followed by a soft support bra worn 24 hours daily for 2 to 3 weeks.

Women who have breast lifts may experience a temporary (up to 6 months) loss of breast and nipple sensation. Breastfeeding is usually not affected. About 20% of women experience capsular contracture.

Breast Reconstruction

With today's advanced surgical procedures, most women who undergo surgery for breast cancer are candidates for breast reconstruction. There are various types of reconstruction, and they are available to women who have had a mastectomy, partial mastectomy, or lumpectomy.

The decision of whether to have breast reconstruction arises at a very emotional time—usually at the same time a woman learns she has breast cancer and needs surgery. It is a time when many questions come up about reconstruction, the most common of which are answered here briefly:

- Is age a factor? As long as a woman is in good general health and chooses a procedure that is compatible with her physical condition, age is usually not a factor. Breast reconstruction is frequently done for women in their 70s.

- Who should not have breast reconstruction? Women who are in poor general health, who have psychological problems that would be exacerbated by the surgery, or who have severe diabetes, Alzheimer's disease, a recent stroke or heart attack, or severe lung disease usually should not have breast reconstruction.

● Do I have to make a decision about having reconstruction before I have the mastectomy? No, but the best time to think about breast reconstruction and to consult with a reconstruction surgeon is before you have your mastectomy. Depending on the type of mastectomy you have, you may be able to undergo immediate reconstruction while you're still on the operating table. There are advantages and disadvantages to having immediate reconstruction (see below). Not all mastectomies lend themselves to this approach, however, which means it is important for you to understand all your options prior to mastectomy. Then if you choose to delay reconstruction, you at least were given the opportunity to make an informed decision.

● Are there any health conditions that could have a negative effect on reconstruction? Women who smoke are more susceptible to postoperative infections and slow healing, so if you smoke it is best to quit before surgery. Obesity is associated with an increased risk of pneumonia, blood clots in the legs, and complications related to anesthesia. The results of both types of reconstruction (implant and flap, both described below) are frequently unsatisfactory in obese women.

● How many operations are involved in breast reconstruction? Most breast reconstructions can be completed in two operations. The majority of the work is done during the first procedure, and the second usually involves reconstructing the nipple and areola, improving symmetry of the breasts, and making any minor adjustments.

● Does breast reconstruction cause cancer? There is no evidence that breast reconstruction causes or contributes to the development of cancer.

• How will my breast reconstruction look in 5 to 10 years? The long-term results of breast reconstruction are different for each woman and depend on the type of procedure you have, your weight, and whether you experience intervening infections or other breast problems.

Choosing a Reconstruction Surgeon

To help you make decisions about breast reconstruction, you will need to select a reconstruction surgeon. Many experts recommend that you interview at least three reconstructive surgeons before you make your choice. Even though you may trust your breast surgeon completely, do not assume the reconstruction surgeon he or she suggests is the one for you. Ask the surgeons how many reconstructions they have performed and how many of each kind (types of reconstruction are discussed below), and if you can talk with patients who have had the surgery you are considering. You need to feel comfortable with the surgeon you choose; all of your questions should be answered completely and patiently. If possible, bring a friend to each interview. Not only can this person offer moral support, but she or he may bring up questions you forget to ask and be a second pair of ears for the information you receive.

Immediate Reconstruction: Yes or No?

Once you know you must undergo mastectomy, it is usually difficult to also have to think about reconstruction. This is the time to surround yourself with supportive individuals, be they family, friends, health care providers, or breast cancer support group members. It is also the time to educate yourself about reconstruction. This is a way to take charge of your health, to have some control over the direction your life is taking.

When it comes to the question of whether you are a candidate for immediate or delayed reconstruction, ask your breast and reconstruction surgeons to explain why they are recommending one or the other. The primary factor that determines the best approach is whether the cancer has affected the lymph nodes and to what extent. Chemotherapy usually is not started until 2 or 3 weeks after mastectomy to allow for healing. If your surgeons believe you must begin chemotherapy immediately to get the best possible outcome, they may recommend delaying reconstruction. Combining mastectomy and reconstruction adds days and occasionally weeks to the healing period, which would significantly delay chemotherapy and possibly have a negative impact on your prognosis.

If your surgeons say immediate reconstruction is an option for you, you must decide if it's best for you. To help you make a decision, it may help to look at the pros and cons (outlined below) and to discuss your concerns with those close to you. The best candidates for immediate reconstruction are women with early breast cancer who are in good general health, women with small breasts, and those who need both breasts reconstructed. However, even if you are ready physically, you may not be mentally or emotionally prepared. In that case, it may be better to delay reconstruction.

Advantages and Disadvantages of Immediate Reconstruction

PROS

- Avoiding an additional surgical procedure.
- One less procedure means less chance of complications.
- Less recovery time needed.
- Costs less money.
- Less time to dwell on the cancer.
- Less negative impact on body image.
- Faster opportunity to get on with your life.

CONS

- Less time to gather information to make an informed decision.
- Surgical procedure is longer, which increases the chances of complications.

- Possible dissatisfaction with the results.
- May delay mourning period for the missing breast.

Breast Reconstruction: Flap or Implant?

A breast can be reconstructed using either a saline implant or a "flap," a procedure that involves using your own skin, fat, and muscle taken from another part of your body. Both approaches have advantages and disadvantages. Implants are performed more often than flap reconstructions: about 60% versus 40% of procedures.

Breast Implants

The implant approach involves surgically inserting a silicone shell filled with a saline (salt) solution into a pocket of muscle at the mastectomy site. (Silicone gel implants, used between 1976 and 1992, have since been all but withdrawn from the market because they are believed to cause connective tissue disorders, such as rheumatoid arthritis, scleroderma, and lupus. See "Breast Augmentation," earlier in this chapter, for further details.) You need enough healthy breast tissue at the surgical site to allow an implant to be placed.

About 70% of women who choose an implant must first have a tissue expander inserted. A tissue expander is an inflatable device that slowly stretches the skin to allow for the eventual insertion of the saline implant. During each of the 6 to 8 weeks that the expander is in place, a small amount of saline is injected into the shell until the temporary implant is about one-third bigger than the desired size. During the next 4 weeks, the breast "settles," and then the expander is replaced by the permanent implant. Both insertion of the expander and placement of the implant can be done on an outpatient basis, and recovery is usually 10 to 14 days.

Flap Reconstruction

There are two types of flap reconstruction. The pedicle, or attached, flap is taken from an area that is close to the breast, usually from the back just below the armpit. The flap remains connected to a muscle stem (the pedicle), which gives it its own blood supply. The flap is stretched, maneuvered into place, and molded to the desired shape. More than 95% of flap procedures performed in the United States use this approach.

A free flap is a section of tissue that is taken from a site completely away from the breast, such as the buttocks. Because all of its blood vessels have been severed, they must be reconnected under a microscope once the flap is in place. Only 3 to 5% of women get a free-flap reconstruction.

The flap procedure that is performed most often is called the TRAM (transverse rectus abdominis myocutaneous), in which the donor skin is taken from the abdomen. It can be done using either the pedicle or free-flap approach. The TRAM allows for reconstruction of larger breasts, and a benefit of this procedure is that women get to lose some excess tissue from their abdomen. Obese women and those with heart disease are generally not good candidates for this procedure.

Which reconstruction approach should you choose? Consult your surgeons and consider the advantages and disadvantages of each surgical approach. Here are some guidelines:

COMPARISON OF RECONSTRUCTION PROCEDURES

	Implant/Expander	*Flap Procedure*
Surgery time	Two operations: each 1.5–2 hours	One 6- to 8-hour operation
Hospitalization	7 days for mastectomy; 1 day when done later	7 to 10 days with or without mastectomy
Aesthetics	Firm, no natural sag, flat across front	Natural shape, very soft

	Implant/Expander	*Flap Procedure*
Common disadvantages	Ripple effect seen through skin; stays the same size if you gain or lose weight	Temporary numbness at donor site; odd sensations while nerves regenerate

Reconstructing the Nipple and Areola

Nearly every mastectomy involves removal of the nipple and areola area. Until recently, reconstruction of the nipple and areola was rarely done, but improved techniques have made this cosmetic change possible. This surgical work is usually done several months after the major reconstruction is completed to allow time for swelling to subside.

A new nipple is usually constructed from the center of the breast using a flap and underlying fat. The procedure can be done on an outpatient basis under local or general anesthesia, and takes 1 to 2 hours. The areola can be done at the same time and may be made from a skin graft. A more popular technique for the areola, however, is tattooing. Because tattoos tend to fade over time, the reconstructed areola will appear darker than the natural one until the new one fades.

Breast Prosthesis

For women who do not choose or who are not suited for breast reconstruction, an external prosthesis is an alternative. A prosthesis can be made of silicone gel inside a plastic shell, or of rubber/latex, foam, or cotton batting. It is typically worn inside a bra tucked into a pocket or attached to the body with tape or special adhesive. Silicone forms, which warm to body temperature and can be matched to your skin tone, are the most expensive. Foam and cotton batting prostheses are the most inexpensive, and can be homemade.

Advantages to having a prosthesis include the following: You avoid a surgical procedure and lengthy recovery time. If you should gain or lose a significant amount of weight after having breast reconstruction, your new breast likely will be a different size than its natural mate. If you have a prosthesis, you can purchase a smaller or larger form to match the existing breast. Disadvantages include worrying that the prosthesis will shift, feeling uncomfortable, and feeling less attractive. Big-breasted women may feel off balance from the weight of the prosthesis, and women who are athletic report that the form can slip during activities and be a source of embarrassment.

Some women elect to use a prosthesis as an interim measure until they are ready, physically and psychologically, to undergo breast reconstruction. The opportunity to wear a prosthesis while they heal gives them a sense of control over their body and a chance to weigh their options.

For more information about breast prostheses, contact the American Cancer Society or visit the Web site for the Michigan Breast Reconstruction Outcome Study (see Resources).

Continuing medical advances are giving women more, better, and safer options when it comes to cosmetic breast surgery; whether it is an elective procedure or a consequence of breast cancer surgery. If you face a decision about cosmetic breast surgery, gather all the information you can about the surgeon, your options, and the procedure. Whatever procedure you choose—or don't choose—should be based on what *you* want and what is safe. In the end, you may decide to do nothing: a small percentage of women (usually those who are very small breasted) say no to reconstruction, no to a prosthesis, and continue living a full life. It is your body; it is your choice.

Glossary

Acini. Glands in the breast that store milk.

Amastia. The absence of one or both nipples.

Areola. The circular pigmented skin that surrounds the nipple.

Atypical hyperplasia. Excessive growth of cells, some of which are abnormal.

Axillary. Referring to the armpit.

Axillary dissection. Surgery to remove the lymph nodes from the armpit.

Baseline mammogram. The first mammogram a woman takes, which is used as a reference point when comparing later mammograms.

Benign. Not cancerous or malignant. A benign growth does not spread (metastasize) to other parts of the body.

Bioflavonoids. A group of water-soluble nutrients that give vegetables and fruits their color. They have anticancer properties.

Biopsy. The use of a needle or scalpel to remove a tissue sample for the purpose of examining it microscopically to determine if it is benign or malignant.

BRCA1 and BRCA2. Breast cancer genes that are associated with familial breast cancer.

Breast augmentation. A surgical procedure to increase the size of a woman's breast. Also called augmentation mammaplasty.

Breast self-examination. An examination of the breasts that women are encouraged to do for themselves each month as a means to screen for breast problems.

Calcifications. Tiny calcium deposits in the breast tissue that are visible on mammography.

Capsular contracture. A shell or mass of scar tissue that often forms as part of the body's reaction to a breast implant.

Carcinogen. A substance that causes cancer.

Chemotherapy. Treatment of cancer using powerful drugs capable of killing cancer cells.

Colostrum. The thick, yellow fluid that is released from the breast during the first 2 to 3 days after giving birth. It contains a high concentration of antibodies, calories, and proteins.

Cyst. A sac that develops in the body that is filled with a liquid or semiliquid material.

Duct. When referring to the female breast, the passageways through which milk travels from the milk glands to reservoirs in the nipple. Most breast cancers are located in the ducts.

Ductal carcinoma in situ (DCIS). Often called a precancerous condition, DCIS is a case in which the cancer cells have not grown beyond their originating point.

Enzyme. A substance that acts as a catalyst to promote chemical reactions in the body without being damaged or destroyed by those reactions.

Estrogen. A type of sex hormone that is produced primarily by the ovaries. There are three kinds of estrogen: estradiol, estrone, and estriol.

Fat necrosis. An area of dead fat that typically is caused by surgery or trauma.

Fibroadenoma. A benign, firm breast tumor most often found in young women.

Fibrocystic breasts. A recurring, cyclic condition in which the breasts are tender, painful, swollen, and lumpy.

Hormone. A chemical produced by the body that can have many functions, including growth, sexual reproduction, and bone development. Estrogen and progesterone are examples of hormones.

Hyperplasia. The excessive growth of cells.

Indole-3-carbinol. A plant chemical found in cruciferous vegetables that helps the body maintain high amounts of good estrogen.

Intraductal. Referring to anything that occurs or is present within the ducts.

Inverted nipple. A nipple that is turned in on itself.

Let-down reflex. The involuntary response of the body that releases the milk from the breast to the infant. Also known as the milk-release reflex.

Lobule.   A small lobe.

Lump.   A mass of tissue; sometimes referred to as a tumor or growth.

Lumpectomy.   The surgical removal of a cancerous lump or tumor along with a small portion of surrounding tissue.

Lymph.   The fluid that flows through the series of vessels called the lymphatic system. Lymph carries various waste products and bacteria, which are filtered through the lymph nodes.

Lymph nodes.   Structures in the lymphatic system that filter out toxins, bacteria, cancer cells, and other waste products.

Macrobiotics.   An Asian philosophy in which eating is based on a balance of yin and yang. The diet consists primarily of brown rice, whole grains, vegetables, fruits, nuts, and legumes.

Malignant.   Cancerous.

Mammogram.   An x-ray of the breast.

Mastectomy.   Surgical removal of the breast.

Mastitis.   A breast infection characterized by pain, inflammation, and swelling.

Mastopexy.   A breast lift.

Metastasis.   Situation in which cancer spreads from one part of the body to another.

Microcalcification.   Tiny calcium deposits in the breast tissue usually detectable on mammography.

Modified radical mastectomy.   Surgical removal of the breast, most of the lymph nodes, and some fat.

Needle aspiration.   A diagnostic tool in which fluid or tissue is removed from a tumor or cyst with a fine needle.

Needle biopsy.   Removal of a tissue sample from the breast using a wide-bore needle and suction.

Oncogenes.   Genes that regulate growth and that can cause tumors to grow.

Organochlorine.   A family of chemicals that are highly carcinogenic to humans, and especially related to breast cancer. DDT is one example.

Oxytocin.   A hormone produced by the pituitary gland that stimulates the release of milk from the breasts.

Palpate.   To feel or examine using the hands.

Pedicle.   A flap of tissue that contains the blood vessels necessary for the tissue to remain viable.

Phytoestrogen.   A plant-based chemical that acts like estrogen and that promotes breast health.

Progesterone.   A female hormone produced by the ovaries during the menstrual cycle.

Progestin.   Synthetic progesterone.

Prolactin.   A hormone produced by the pituitary gland that promotes lactation and growth of both healthy and cancerous breast cells.

Prostaglandins.   Hormone-like substances that have various impacts on organ function.

Radical mastectomy.   Removal of the breast, the underlying muscles, and the lymph nodes under the arm.

Sentinel node biopsy.   A procedure in which only one or a few of the first nodes in the axillary are removed through a small incision.

Simple mastectomy.   Surgical removal of the breast only while retaining the muscle and lymph nodes.

Skin-sparing mastectomy.   A procedure in which the breast is removed using smaller incisions and less skin is cut away.

Tamoxifen (Nolvadex).   An estrogen-blocker drug often prescribed as an alternative to chemotherapy in postmenopausal women. It reportedly helps protect against breast cancer.

Tissue expander.   An implant that can be inflated to expand the breast tissue and prepare it for the permanent implant.

TRAM breast reconstruction.   Breast reconstruction in which the transverse rectus abdominis myocutaneous (TRAM) flap is used to build a breast.

Tumor.   An abnormal growth of tissue that can be malignant or benign.

Ultrasound.   A diagnostic technique that uses high-frequency sound waves to generate images.

Xenoestrogen.   An estrogen-like substance that exists in the environment and can cause powerful estrogenic reactions in the body. Examples include pesticides, air pollutants, secondhand smoke, and cleaning chemicals.

Sources

Chapter 1

Epstein, Samuel S., and David Steinman. *The Breast Cancer Prevention Program*. New York: Macmillan, 1997.

Lauersen, Niels H., and Eileen Stukane. *The Complete Book of Breast Care*. New York: Ballantine, 1996.

Love, Susan M., *Dr. Susan Love's Breast Book*, 2nd ed. Reading, MA: Addison-Wesley Publishing, 1995.

Stanway, A., and P. Stanway. *The Breast*. London: Granada Publishing, 1982.

Chapter 2

Anderson, J. W., et al. Breast-feeding and cognitive development: A meta-analysis. *American Journal of Clinical Nutrition* 1999 Oct; 70(4):525–535.

Birnbaum, C. S., et al. Serum concentrations of antidepressants and benzodiazepines in nursing infants. A case series. *Pediatrics* 1999 July; 104(1):e11.

Chisholm C.A., and J. A. Kuller. A guide to the safety of CNS active agents during breastfeeding. *Drug Safety* 1997 Aug; 17(2):127–142.

Coogan, Patricia, et al. Lactation and breast carcinoma risk in South African population. *Cancer* 1999; 86:982–989.

Cunningham, Allan S. *Breastfeeding, Bottle-feeding and Illness: An Annotated Bibliography*. Lactation Resource Center, Nursing Mother's Association of Australia, 1986.

Drane, D. Breastfeeding and formula feeding: a preliminary economic analysis. *Breastfeed Ref* 1997; 5:7–15.

Enger, S.M., et al. Breastfeeding history, pregnancy experience, and risk of breast cancer. *British Journal of Cancer* 1997; 76(1):118–123.

Freudenheim, J.L., et al. Lactation history and breast cancer risk. *American Journal of Epidemiology* 1997 Dec. 1; 146(11):932–998.

Gliksman, Michele Isaacs, and Theresa Foy DiGeronimo. *The Complete Idiot's Guide to Pregnancy and Childbirth*. New York: Macmillan, 1999.

Goyco, P.G., and R.C. Beckerman. Sudden infant death syndrome. *Current Problems in Pediatrics* 1990; 20:299–346; cited in the National SIDS Resource Center Information Sheet #1.

Gwinn, M. L. Pregnancy, breast feeding and oral contraceptives and the risk of epithelial ovarian cancer. *Journal of Clinical Epidemiology* 1990; 43:559–568.

Hahn-Soric, M., et al. Antibody responses to parenteral and oral vaccines are impaired by conventional low-protein formulas as compared to breast-feeding. *Acta Paediatrica Scandinavica* 1990; 79:1137–1142.

Haller, C.A., et al. Breastfeeding. 1999 perspective. *Current Opinions in Pediatrics* 1999 Oct; 11(5):379–383.

Horwood J. L., and D. M. Fergusson. Breastfeeding and later cognitive and academic outcomes. *Pediatrics* 1998 Jan; 101(1):E9.

Howie, P. W., et al. Protective effect of breast feeding against infection. *British Medical Journal* 1990; 300:11–16.

Hreschyshyn, M. M., et al. Associations of parity, breast-feeding and birth control pills with lumbar spine and femoral neck bone densities. *American Journal of Obstetrics and Gynecology* 1988; 159:318–322.

Kalwart, H. J., and B. L. Specker. Bone mineral loss during lactation and recovery after weaning. *Obstetrics and Gynecology* 1995; 86:26–32.

Lee, Nikki. Benefits of breastfeeding and their economic impact: a report. August 1977. Available from the author at Nursing Mothers Advisory Council, www.nursingmoms.net.

Levine, L. L., and N. T. Ilowite. Sclerodermalike esophageal disease in children breastfed by mothers with silicone breast implants. *Journal of the American Medical Association* 1994; 271:213–216.

Lucas, et al. Early diet of preterm infants and development of allergic or atopic disease: randomized prospective study. *British Medical Journal* 1990; 300:387.

Nayak, N., et al. Specific secretory IgA in the milk of *Giardia lamblia*–infected and uninfected women. *Journal of Infectious Diseases* 1987 Apr; 155(4):724–727.

Neifert, Marianne. *Dr. Mom's Guide to Breastfeeding*. New York: Penguin, 1998.

Newcomb, P.A., et al. Lactation in relation to postmenopausal breast cancer. *American Journal of Epidemiology* 1999 Jul 15; 150(2):174–182.

Pisacane, A., et al. Breastfeeding and acute lower respiratory infection. *Acta Paediatrica* 1994; 83:714–718.

Rosenblatt, K. A., et al. Lactation and the risk of epithelial ovarian cancer. The WHO collaborative study of neoplasia and steroid contraceptives. *International Journal of Epidemiology* 1993 Apr; 22(2):192–197.

Chapter 4

American Institute for Cancer Research and the World Cancer Research Fund. *Food, Nutrition, and the Prevention of Cancer: A Global Perspective.* December 1997.

Berma, S. P., et al. The inhibition of the estrogenic effects of pesticides and environmental chemicals by curcumin and isoflavonoids. *Environmental Health Perspectives* 1998 Dec; 106(12):807–812.

Challier, B., et al. Garlic, onion and cereal fibre as protective factors for breast cancer: A French case-control study. *European Journal of Epidemiology* 1998 Dec; 14(8):737–747.

Chang, Y. C., et al. Cytostatic and antiestrogenic effects of 2-(indol-3-ylmethyl)-3,3'-diindolylmethane, a major in vivo product of dietary indole-3-carbinol. *Biochemical Pharmacology* 1999 Sep 1; 59(5):825–834.

Cover, C. M., et al. Indole-3-carbinol and tamoxifen cooperate to arrest the cell cycle of MCF-7 human breast cancer cells. *Cancer Research* 1999 Mar 15; 59(6):1244–1251.

DeStefani, E., et al. Dietary fiber and risk of breast cancer: A case-control study in Uruguay. *Nutrition and Cancer* 1997; 28(1):14–19.

Fotsis, T., et al. Phytoestrogens and inhibition of angiogenesis. *Baillieres Clinical Endocrinology and Metabolism* 1998 Dec; 12(4):649–666.

John, E. M. Vitamin D and breast cancer risk: The NHANESI epidemiologic follow-up study, 1971–1975 to 1992. *Cancer Epidemiology Biomarkers and Prevention.*

La Vecchia, C., et al. Fibers and breast cancer risk. *Nutrition and Cancer* 1997; 28(3):264–269.

Li, Y., et al. Induction of apoptosis and inhibition of c-erbB-2 in MDA-MB-435 cells by genistein. *International Journal of Oncology* 1999 Sept; 15(3):525–533.

Milo, L., et al. Lutein and zeaxanthin inhibit human breast cancer cell proliferation. *FASEB Journal* 1998; 12:A830 (Abstract 4810).

Position of the American Dietetic Association: function foods. *Journal of the American Dietetic Association* 1999; 99:1278.

Rose, D. P., and J. M. Connolly. Omega-3 fatty acids as cancer chemopreventive agents. *Pharmacology Therapy* 1999 Sept; 83(3):217–244.

Shao, Z. M., et al. Genistein exerts multiple suppressive effects on human breast carcinoma cells. *Cancer Research* 1998 Nov. 1; 58(21):4851–4857.

Sharoni, Y., et al. Effects of lycopene enriched tomato oleoresin on 7,12-dimethyl-benz(1)anthracene-induced rat mammary tumors. *Cancer Detection and Prevention* 1997; 21(2):118–123.

Verma, S. P., et al. Curcumin and genistein, plant natural products, show synergistic inhibitory effects on the growth of human breast cancer MCF-7 cells induced by estrogenic pesticides. *Biochemical and Biophysical Research Communications* 1997 Apr 28; 233(3):692–696.

Wargovich, M. J. Experimental evidence for cancer preventive elements in foods. *Cancer Letter* 1997 Mar 19; 114(1-2):11–17.

Chapter 5

Breast cancer and pesticides. *Soil and Health*, January 1994.

Brenner, et al. The antiproliferative effect of vitamin D analogs on MCF-human breast cancer cells. *Cancer Letter* 1995; 92(1):77–82.

Clark, L., et al. Effects of selenium supplementation for cancer prevention in patients with carcinoma of the skin. *Journal of the American Medical Association* 1996; 276:1957–1963.

Combs, G. F., et al. Emerging relationships of vitamins and cancer risks. *Current Opinion in Clinical Nutritional Metabolism Care* 1998 Nov; 1(6):519–523.

de Blasio, F., et al. N-acetyl cysteine (NAC) in preventing nausea and vomiting induced by chemotherapy in patients suffering from inoperable non small cell lung cancer (NSCLC). *Chest* 1996; 110(4, suppl):103S.

Dorgan, J. F., et al. Relationships of serum carotenoids, retinol, alpha-tocopherol, and selenium with breast cancer risk. Results from a prospective study in Columbia, Missouri. *Cancer Causes and Control* 1998 Jan; 9(1):89–97.

Duda, R. B., et al. American ginseng and breast cancer therapeutic agents synergistically inhibit MCF-7 breast cancer cell growth. *Journal of Surgical Oncology* 1999 Dec; 72(4):230–239.

Folkers, K., and A. Wolaniuk. Research on coenzyme Q10 in clinical medicine and in immunomodulation. *Drugs Under Experimental and Clinical Research* 1985; 11:539–545.

Gaynor, Mitchell L., and Jerry Hickey. *Dr. Gaynor's Cancer Prevention Program.* New York: Kensington Books, 1999.

Halaska, M., et al. Treatment of cyclical mastodynia using an extract of vitex agnus castus: results of a double-blind comparison with a placebo. *Ceskoslovenska Gynekologica* 1998 Oct; 63(5):388–392.

Jolliet, P., et al. Plasma coenzyme Q10 concentrations in breast cancer: prognosis and therapeutic consequences. *International Journal of Clinical Pharmacology and Therapeutics* 1998 Sep; 36(9):506–509.

Joshi, S. S., et al. Cytotoxic effects of a novel grape seed proanthrocyanidin extract on cultured human cancer cells. *Scientific Proceedings of the 89th Annual Meeting of the American Association for Cancer Research* 1998 Mar; vol. 39.

Komori, et al. Anticarcinogenic activity of green tea polyphenols. *Japanese Journal of Clinical Oncology* 1993; 23(3):186–190.

Lipkin, M., and H. L. Newmark. Vitamin D, calcium and prevention of breast cancer: a review. *Journal of the American College of Nutrition* 1999 Oct; 18(suppl 5):392S–397S.

Lockwood, K., et al. Partial and complete regression of breast cancer in patients in relation to dosage of coenzyme Q10. *Biochemical and Biophysical Research Communications* 1994 Mar 30; 199(3):1504–1508.

Meyer, K., et al. *Zingiber officinale* (ginger) used to prevent 8-Mop associated nausea. *Dermatologic Nursing* 1995; 7:242–244.

Myers, C., W. McGuire, and R. Young. Adriamycin amelioration of toxicity by alpha-tocopherol. *Cancer Treatment Report* 1976; 60:961–962.

Perez Ripoll, E. A., et al. Vitamin E enhances the chemotherapeutic effects of adriamycin on human prostatic carcinoma cells in vitro. *Journal of Urology* 1986; 136:529–531.

Singletary, K., et al. Inhibition by rosemary and carnosol of 7,1-dimethyl-benz[a]anthracene (DMBA)-induced rat mammary tumorigenesis and in vivo DMBA-DNA adduct formation. *Cancer Letter* 1996 June 24; 104(1):43–48.

Wadleigh, R. G., et al. Vitamin E in the treatment of chemotherapy-induced mucositis. *American Journal of Medicine* 1992; 92:481–484.

Wong, G. Y., et al. Dose-ranging study of indole-3-carbinol for breast cancer prevention. *Journal of Cellular Biochemistry* 1997; Suppl 28–29: 111–116.

Wood, L. A. Possible prevention of Adriamycin-induced alopecia by tocopherol. *New England Journal of Medicine* 1985; 312:1060 (letter).

Zava, D. T., et al. Estrogen and progestin bioactivity of foods, herbs, and spices. *Proceedings of the Society for Experimental Biology and Medicine* 1998 Mar; 217(3):369–378.

Zhang, S., et al. Dietary carotenoids and vitamins A, C, and E and risk of breast cancer. *Journal of the National Cancer Institute* 1999 Mar 17; 91(6):547–556.

Chapter 6

Anonymous. Norplant update. *Breast Implants* 1995; 3(8):1–3.

Asbell, B. *The Pill: A Biography of the Drug That Changed the World.* New York: Random House, 1995, p. 305.

Berrino, F., et al. Serum sex hormone levels after menopause and subsequent breast cancer risk. *Journal of the National Cancer Institute* 1996; 88(5):291–296.

Cancer and Steroid Hormone Study of the Centers for Disease Control and the National Institute of Child Health and Human Development. Oral contraceptive use and the risk of breast cancer. *New England Journal of Medicine* 1986; 315:405–411.

Chang, K., et al. Influences of percutaneous administration of estradiol and progesterone on human breast epithelial cell cycle in vivo. *Fertility and Sterility* 1995; 63(4):785–791.

Collaborative Group on Hormonal Factors in Breast Cancer. Breast cancer and hormonal contraceptives: further results. *Contraception* 1996 Sep; 54(suppl 3):1S–106S.

De Lignieres, B. Oral micronized progesterone. *Clinical Therapeutics* 1999 Jan; 21(1):41–60.

International Agency for Research on Cancer. *Sex Hormones.* Lyon, France: World Health Organization, IARC monograph, 1979; 21:485.

Kavanagh, A. Hormone replacement therapy and accuracy of mammographic screening. *Lancet* 2000 Jan 22; 355:270–274.

Lee, John R. Osteoporosis reversal: the role of progesterone. *Internal Clinical Nutrition Reviews* 1990; 10(3).

Potashnik, G., et al. Fertility drugs and the risk of breast and ovarian cancer: results of a long-term follow-up study. *Fertility and Sterility* 1999 May; 71(5):853–859.

Ricci, E., et al. Fertility drugs and the risk of breast cancer. *Human Reproduction* 1999 Jun; 14(6):1653–1655.

Romieu, I., J.A. Berlin, and G. Colditz. Oral contraceptives and breast cancer: review and meta-analysis. *Cancer* 1990 Dec 1; 66(11):2253–2263.

Ross, R., et al. Effect of hormone replacement therapy on breast cancer risk: estrogen versus estrogen plus progestin. *Journal of the National Cancer Institute* 2000 Feb 16; 92(4):328–332.

Schairer, C., et al. Menopausal estrogen and estrogen-progestin replacement therapy and breast cancer risk. *Journal of the American Medical Association* 2000 Jan 26; 283:485–491.

Schneider, D. L., et al. Timing of postmenopausal estrogen for optimal bone mineral density. The Rancho Bernardo study. *Journal of the American Medical Association*. 1997; 227(1):543–547.

Seaman, Barbara. *The Doctor's Case Against the Pill*. Alameda, CA: Hunter House, 1995 (originally published 1969).

Skegg, D. C., et al. Depo medroxyprogesterone acetate and breast cancer. A pooled analysis of the World Heath Organization and New Zealand studies. *Journal of the American Medical Association* 1995; 273(10):799–804.

Ursin, G., et al. Use of oral contraceptives and risk of breast cancer in young women. *Breast Cancer Research and Treatment* 1998 Jul; 50(2):175–184.

Chapter 7

Albanes, D., et al. Physical activity and risk of cancer in the NHANES I population. *American Journal of Public Health* 1989; 79(6):744–750.

Andersen, B., et al. Stress and immune response after surgical treatment for regional breast cancer. *Journal of the National Cancer Institute* 1998 Jan 7; 90(1):30–36.

Berstein, L., et al. Physical exercise and reduced risk of breast cancer in young women. *Journal of the National Cancer Institute* 1994; 86:1403–1408.

Brennan, C., and J. Stevens. A grounded theory approach towards understanding the self-perceived effects of meditation on people being treated for cancer. *Australian Journal of Holistic Nursing* 1998; 5(2):20–26.

Chen, C.C., et al. Adverse life events and breast cancer: case-control study. *British Medical Journal* 1995 Dec 9; 311(7019):1527–1530.

Frisch, R. E., et al. Lower prevalence of breast cancer and cancers of the reproductive system among college athletes compared to nonathletes. *British Journal of Cancer* 1985; 52:885–891.

Frisch, R. E., et al. Lower lifetime occurrence of breast cancer and cancers of the reproductive system among former college athletes. *American Journal of Clinical Nutrition* 1987; 45:328–335.

Gimbel, M. A. Yoga, meditation, and imagery: clinical applications. *Nurse Practitioner Forum* 1998 Dec; 9(4):243–255.

Gray, R., et al. A qualitative study of breast cancer self-help groups. *Psychooncology* 1997 Dec; 6(4):279–289.

Kolcaba, K., and C. Fox. The effects of guided imagery on comfort of women with early stage breast cancer undergoing radiation therapy. *Oncology Nursing Forum* 1999 Jan–Feb; 26(1):67–72.

Pilisuk, M., et al. Participant assessment of a nomedical breast cancer support group. *Alternative Therapies in Health and Medicine* 1997 Sep; 3(5):72–80.

Protheroe, D., et al. Stressful life events and difficulties and onset of breast cancer: case control study. *British Medical Journal* 1999 Oct. 16; 319(7216):1027–1030.

Roberts, F. D., et al. Self-reported stress and risk of breast cancer. *Cancer* 1996 Mar 15; 77(6):1089–1093

Rona, Zoltan, ed. *Encyclopedia of Natural Healing*. Blaine, WA: Natural Life Publishing, 1997.

Shrock, D., et al. Effects of a psychosocial intervention on survival among patients with stage I breast and prostate cancer: a matched case-control study. *Alternative Therapies in Health and Medicine* 1999 May; 5(3):49–55.

Spiegel, D., and R. Moore. Imagery and hypnosis in the treatment of cancer patients. *Oncology* 1997 Aug; 11(8):1179–1189.

Walker, L. G., et al. Psychological, clinical and pathological effects of relaxation training and guided imagery during primary chemotherapy. *British Journal of Cancer* 1999 Apr; 80(1–2):262–268.

Warren, M. P. The effects of exercise on pubertal progression and reproductive function in girls. *Journal of Clinical Endocrinology and Metabolism* 1989; 51(5):1150–1157.

Chapter 8

Digital mammography: Why hasn't it been approved for US hospitals? *Health Devices* 2000 Jan; 28(1):14–21.

Edell, S. L., and M. D. Eisen. Current imaging modalities for the diagnosis of breast cancer. *Del Medical Journal* 1999 Sep; 71(9):377–382.

Elwood, J. M., et al. The effectiveness of breast cancer screening by mammography in younger women. *Online Journal of Current Clinical Trials* 1993 Feb 25; 2:32.

Harms, S. E., et al. MR imaging of the breast: current status and future potential. *American Journal of Roentgenology* 1994; 163:1039–1047.

Jones, B.F. A reappraisal of the use of infrared thermal image analysis in medicine. *IEEE Transactions on Medical Imaging* 1998 Dec; 17(6): 1019–1027.

Khalkhali, I., et al. Review of imaging techniques for the diagnosis of breast cancer: a new role of prone scintimammography using technetium-99m sestamibi. *European Journal of Nuclear Medicine* 1994; 21:357–362.

Khalkhali, I., et al. The usefulness of scintimammography (SMM) in patients with dense breasts on mammogram. *Journal of Nuclear Medicine* 1995; 36:52.

Khalkhali, I., et al. Scintimammography: the new role of technetium-99m sestamibi imaging for the diagnosis of breast carcinoma. *Quarterly Journal of Nuclear Medicine* 1997 Sep; 41(3):231–238.

Reynolds, H. E. Advances in breast imaging. *Hematology-Oncology Clinics of North America* 1999 Apr; 13(2):333–348.

Taber, L. et al. The natural history of breast carcinoma: what have we learned from screening? *Cancer* 1999 Aug 1; 86(3): 449–462.

Tiling, R., et al. Role of technetium-99m sestamibi scintimammography and contrast-enhanced magnetic resonance imaging for the evaluation of indeterminate mammograms. *European Journal of Nuclear Medicine* 1997 Oct; 24(10):1221–1229.

Chapter 9

American Institute for Cancer Research's Program for Cancer Prevention. *Stopping Cancer Before It Starts*. New York: Golden Books, 1999.

Aschengrau, A., and D. M. Ozonoff. *Upper Cape Cancer Incidence Study. Final Report*. Boston: Boston University School of Public Health, September 1991.

Bhatta, S., et al. Breast cancer and other second neoplasms after childhood Hodgkin's disease. *New England Journal of Medicine* 1996; 334(12):745–751.

Boorman, G. A., et al. Effect of 25 week magnetic field exposure in a DMBA initiation-promotion mammary gland model in Sprague Dawley rats. *Carcinogenesis* 1999 May; 20(5):899–904.

Boorman, G. A., et al. Chronic toxicity/oncogenicity evaluation of 60 Hz (power frequency) magnetic fields in F344/N rats. *Toxicologic Pathology* 1999 May–Jun; 27(3):267–278.

Boyer, Andrea P., et al. Recommendations for the prevention of chronic disease: the application for breast disease. *American Journal of Clinical Nutrition* 1988; 48:896–900.

Brotons, J. A., et al. Xenoestrogens released from lacquer coatings in food cans. *Environmental Health Perspectives* 1995 Jun; 103(6):608–612.

Burley, V. J. Sugar consumption and human cancer in sites other than the digestive tract. *European Journal of Cancer Prevention* 1998 Aug; 7(4):253–277.

Calle E. E., et al. Cigarette smoking and risk of fatal breast cancer. *American Journal of Epidemiology* 1994 May 15; 139(10):1001–1007.

Calle, E. E., et al. Occupation and breast cancer mortality in a prospective cohort of US women. *American Journal of Epidemiology* 1998 Jul 15; 148(2):191–197.

Cohen, L. A., et al. Dietary fat and mammary cancer I. Promoting effect of dietary fats and N-nitrosomethylurea-induced rat mammary tumorigenesis. *Journal of the National Cancer Institute* 1986; 77:33–42.

Committee on Diet, Nutrition and Cancer. *Diet, Nutrition and Cancer.* Washington, DC: National Academy Press, 1982.

Consumers Union. Letter from Edward Groth III and Mark Silbergeld to FDA (Joseph Levitt) 5 June 1998. Can be seen at www.consumer.org%2Ffood%Fplasticny698.htm.

Coogan, P. F., et al. Variation in female breast cancer risk by occupation. *American Journal of Industrial Medicine* 1996 Oct; 30(4):430–437.

Dees, C., S. Garrett, C. D. Henley, and C. Travis. Effects of 60-Hz fields, estradiol and xenoestrogens on human breast cancer cells. *Radiation Research* 1996 Oct; 146(4): 444–452.

Environmental Protection Agency. *Journal of Pesticide Reform,* Spring 1988: 29.

Environmental Working Group and the Nutrition Action Health Letter 24 (1997): 7, Center for Science in the Public Interest.

Epstein, S. Potential public health hazards of biosynthetic milk hormones. *International Journal of Health Services* 1990; 20:73–84.

Epstein, S. S. Unlabeled milk from cows treated with biosynthetic growth hormones: a case of regulatory abdication. *International Journal of Health Services* 1996; 26(1):1730–1785.

Falck, F, A. Ricci, M. S. Wolff, et al. Pesticides and polychlorinated biphenyl residues in human breast lipids and their relation to breast cancer. *Archives of Environmental Health* 47 (1992):143–146.

Favero A., M. Parpinel, and S. Frandeschi. Diet and risk of breast cancer: major findings from an Italian case-control study. *Biomedical Pharmacotherapy* 1998; 52(3):109–115.

Feychting, M., and A. Ahlbom. Magnetic fields and cancer in people residing near Swedish high-voltage power lines. *American Journal of Epidemiology* 1993; 183(7):467–481.

Goldin, Barry R., et al. Effect of diet on the plasma levels, metabolism and excretion of estrogens. *American Journal of Clinical Nutrition* 1988; 48:787–790.

Hankinson, Susan E., et al. Circulating concentrations of insulin-like growth factor I and risk of breast cancer. *The Lancet* 1998; 351: 1393–1396.

Harvard Center for Cancer Prevention. *Harvard Report on Cancer Prevention, Volume 1: Causes of Human Cancer. Cancer Causes and Control* 1996 (suppl).

Heath, C. W. Electromagnetic field exposure and cancer: a review of epidemiologic evidence. *CA: A Cancer Journal for Clinicians* 1996; 46(1): 29–44.

Herman, Marcia E. Secondary sexual characteristics and menses in young girls seen in office practice: a study from the Pediatric Research in Office

Settings Network, *Pediatrics* 1999; 99:505–512.

Howe, G. R., et al. Dietary factors and risk of breast cancer: combined analysis of 12 case-control studies. *Journal of the National Cancer Institute* 1990; 82:561–569.

Iknayan, H. F. Carcinoma associated with irradiation of the mature breast. *Radiation* 1975; 114:431–433.

Jacobs, M. M. *Exercise, Calories, Fat, and Cancer.* New York: Plenum Press, 1996.

Janower, M., and O. Miettinen. Neoplasms after childhood irradiation of the thymus gland. *Journal of the American Medical Association* 1971; 215:753–756.

Katan, Grundy, and Willett. Should a low-fat, high-carbohydrate diet by recommended for everyone? Beyond low-fat diets. *New England Journal of Medicine* 1997 Aug 21; 337(8):563–566.

Kelsey, Jennifer L., et al. Epidemiology and prevention of breast cancer. *Annual Reviews of Public Health* 1996; 17:47–67.

Levy, S., et al. Correlation of stress factors with sustained depression of natural killer cell activity and predicted prognosis in patients with breast cancer. *Journal of Clinical Oncology* 1987 Mar; 5(3):348–353.

Loberg, L. I., et al. Gene expression in human breast epithelial cells exposed to 60Hz magnetic fields. *Carcinogenesis* 1999 Aug; 20(8):1633–1636.

MacKenzie, I. Breast cancer following multiple fluoroscopies. *British Journal of Cancer* 1965; 19:1–8.

McKenna, M. C., et al. Psychosocial factors and the development of breast cancer: a meta-analysis. *Health Psychology* 1999 Sep; 18:520–531.

Minton, J. P., et al. Response of fibrocystic disease to caffeine withdrawal and correlation of cyclic nucleotides with breast disease. *American Journal of Obstetrics and Gynecology* 1979; 135:157–158.

Modan, B., et al. Increased risk of breast cancer after low-dose radiation. *The Lancet* 1989; 629–631.

Morabia, A., et al. Relation of breast cancer with passive and active exposure to tobacco smoke. *American Journal of Epidemiology* 1996 May 1; 143(9):918–928.

New York State Department of Health. *Residence Near Industries and High Traffic Areas and the Risk of Breast Cancer on Long Island, April 1994.* Division of Occupational Health and Environmental Epidemiology.

Prentice, Ross, et al. Dietary fat and cancer: consistency of the epidemiologic data, and disease prevention that may follow from a practical reduction in fat consumption. *Cancer Causes and Control* 1990; 1:81–97.

Rachel's Environmental Weekly #555, Environmental Research Foundation, P.O. Box 5036, Annapolis, MD 21403; dioxin in chicken.

Reichman, Marsha, et al. Effects of alcohol consumption on plasma and urinary hormone concentrations in premenopausal women. *Journal of the National Cancer Institute* 1993; 85:722–727.

Rohan, T. E. Cigarette smoking and risk of benign proliferative epithelial disorders of the breast. *European Journal of Epidemiology* 1999 Jul; 15(6):529–535.

Schechter, M. T., et al. Cigarette smoking and breast cancer: case-control studies of prevalent and incident cancer in the Canadian National Breast Screening Study. *American Journal of Epidemiology* 1989 Aug; 130(2):213–220.

Seely, S., and D. F. Horrobin. Diet and breast cancer: the possible connection with sugar consumption. *Medical Hypothesis* 1983; 11(3):319–327.

Shafer, N., and R. W. Shafer. Potential of carcinogenic effects of hair dyes. *New York State Journal of Medicine* 1976; 76:394–396.

Shore, R. E., et al. Breast neoplasms in women treated with x-rays for acute postpartum mastitis. *Journal of the National Cancer Institute* 1977; 59(3):813–822.

Shore, R. E., et al. Synergism between radiation and other risk factors for breast cancer. *Preventive Medicine* 1980; 9:815–822.

Smith-Warner, S. A., et al. Alcohol and breast cancer in women: a pooled analysis of cohort studies. *Journal of the American Medical Association* 18 Feb. 1998; 279(7):535–540.

Spiegel, D., et al. Effect of psychosocial treatment on survival of patients with metastatic breast cancer. *The Lancet* 14 Oct 1989; 2(8668):888–891.

Swanson, C.A., et al. Alcohol consumption and breast cancer risk among women under age 45 years. *Epidemiology* 1997 May; 8(3):231–237.

Swift, M. Ionizing radiation, breast cancer, and ataxia-telangiectasia. *Journal of the National Cancer Institute* 1994; 86(21):1571–1572.

Tannenbaum, A., et al. Nutrition in relation to cancer. *Advances in Cancer Research* 1953; 1:451–465

Tavani, A., A. Pregnolato, C. La Vecchia, et al. Coffee consumption and the risk of breast cancer. *European Journal of Cancer Prevention* Feb 1998; 7(1):77–82.

Thomas, David B., and Margaret K. Karagas. *Cancer Epidemiology and Prevention* 2nd ed. New York: Oxford University Press, 1996, pp. 236–254.

Tseng, M., et al. Calculation of population attributable risk for alcohol and breast cancer (United States). *Cancer Causes and Control* 1999 Apr; 10(2):119–123.

Upton, A. C., et al., eds. *Radiation Carcinogenesis.* New York: Elsevier, 1986.

Wertheimer, N. and E. Leeper. Magnetic field exposure related to cancer subtypes. *Annals of the New York Academy of Sciences* 1987; 502:43–54.

Willett, W. C., et al. Dietary fat and fiber in relation to risk of breast cancer. An 8-year follow-up. *Journal of the American Medical Association* 1992 Oct 21; 268(15):2037–2044.

Wolff, M. S., P. G. Toniolo, E. W. Lee, et al. Blood levels of organochlorine residues and risk of breast cancer. *Journal of the National Cancer Institute* 1993; 85:648–662.

Wolff, M. S., and A. Weston. Breast cancer risk and environmental exposures. *Environmental Health Perspectives* 1997 Jun; 105 (suppl 4):891–896.

Wolk, A., et al. A prospective study of association of monounsaturated fat and other types of fat with risk of breast cancer. *Archives of Internal Medicine* 12 Jan 1998; 158(1):41–45.

Wu, A. H., M. C. Pike, and D. O. Stram. Meta-analysis: dietary fat intake, serum estrogen levels, and the risk of breast cancer. *Journal of the National Cancer Institute* 1999 Mar. 17; 91(6): 529–534.

Zhang, Y. et al. Alcohol consumption and risk of breast cancer: the Framingham Study revisited. *American Journal of Epidemiology* 15 Jan 1999; 149(2):93–101.

Chapter 10

American Institute for Cancer Research. *Stopping Cancer Before It Starts.* New York: Golden Books, 1999.

Colditz, G. A. Type of post-menopausal hormone use and risk of breast cancer: 12-year follow up from the Nurses' Health Study. *Cancer Causes and Control* 1992 Sep; 3:433–439.

A Consideration of the Potential of Silicone to Cause Cancer in Humans. Report by Dr. Tom Withrow based on internal FDA review. 9 August 1988.

Epstein, Samuel, and David Steinman. *The Breast Cancer Prevention Program.* New York: Macmillan, 1997.

General and plastic surgery devices: effective data of requirement for premarket approval of silicone gel-filled breast prosthesis. *Federal Register* 1990; 55(90):20,568–20,577.

Huang, Z., et al. Dual effects of weight and weight gain on breast cancer risk. *Journal of the American Medical Association* 1997 Nov 5; 278(17):1407–1411.

Keon, Joseph. *The Truth About Breast Cancer.* Mill Valley, CA: Parissound, 1999.

Lauersen, Niels H., and Eileen Stukane. *The Complete Book of Breast Care.* New York: Fawcett, 1996.

La Vecchia, C. et al. Body mass index and post-menopausal breast cancer: an age-specific analysis. *British Journal of Cancer* 1997; 75(3):441–444.

Lee, M. M., et al. Alternative therapies used by women with breast cancer in four ethnic populations. *Journal of the National Cancer Institute* 2000 Jan. 5; 92(1):42–47.

Limin, L., et al. The TSG101 tumor susceptibility gene is located in chromosome 11 band p15 and is mutated in human breast cancer. *Cell* 1997; 88:143–154.

Magnusson, C., et al. Body size in different periods of life and breast cancer risk in post-menopausal women. *International Journal of Cancer* 1998 Mar 30; 76(1):29–34.

Potter, M., et al. Induction of plasmocytomas with silicone gel in genetically susceptible strains of mice. *Journal of the National Cancer Institute* 1994; 86(14):1058–1065.

West, M. M., and S. A. Joselyn. Racial differences in breast carcinoma survival. *Cancer* 2000 Jan 1; 88:114–123.

Chapter 11

Ader, D. N., et al. Cyclical mastalgia: premenstrual syndrome or recurrent pain disorder? *Journal of Psychosomatic Obstetrics and Gynaecology* 1999 Dec; 20(4):198–202.

American Cancer Society. http://www.acs.org.

Berger, Karen, and John Bostwick, III. *A Woman's Decision: Breast Care, Treatment and Reconstruction.* New York: St. Martin's, 1998.

Boyd, N. F., V. McGuire, and P. Shannon. Effect of a low-fat high-carbohydrate diet on symptoms of cyclical mastopathy. *The Lancet* 1988; 2:128–132.

Isaacs, H. J. Benign tumors of the breast. *Obstetrics and Gynecology* 1994; 21:487–497.

Lauersen, Niels H., and Eileen Stukane. *The Complete Book of Breast Care.* New York: Fawcett, 1996.

Understanding Breast Changes: A Health Guide for All Women. Pub. #97–336. Washington, DC: National Cancer Institute, 1997.

Chapter 12

American Cancer Society. http://www.cancer.org.

American Society of Plastic Reconstructive Surgeons. www.asprs.org.

Berger, Karen, and John Bostwick, III. *A Woman's Decision: Breast Care, Treatment and Reconstruction.* New York: St. Martin's, 1998.

Michigan Breast Reconstruction Outcome Study. www.surg.med.umich.edu/plastic/breastrecon/brhtml.

National Alliance of Breast Cancer Organizations fact sheets. http://www.nabco.org.

National Cancer Institute. http://www.cancernet.nci.nih.gov.

Resources

For Further Reading

Altman, Roberta. *Every Woman's Handbook for Preventing Cancer.* New York: Pocket Books, 1996.

American Institute for Cancer Research. *Stopping Cancer Before It Starts.* New York: Golden Books, 1999.

Asbell, B. *The Pill: A Biography of the Drug That Changed the World.* New York: Random House, 1995.

Berger, Karen, and John Boswick, III. *A Woman's Decision: Breast Care, Treatment and Reconstruction.* 3rd ed. New York: St. Martin's Griffin, 1998.

Bragg, Ginna Bell, and David Simon. *A Simple Celebration: A Vegetarian Cookbook for Body, Mind and Spirit.* New York: Harmony, 1997.

Carson, Rachel. *Silent Spring.* Boston: Houghton Mifflin, 1962.

Eiger, Marvin S., and Sally Wendkosolds. *The Complete Book of Breastfeeding.* New York: Workman Publishing, 1999.

Epstein, Samuel S., and David Steinman. *The Breast Cancer Prevention Program.* New York: Macmillan, 1997.

Erasmus, Udo. *Fats That Heal, Fats That Kill.* Rev. ed. Burnaby, BC, Canada: Alive Books, 1999.

Fox, Nicols. *Spoiled: The Dangerous Truth About a Food Chain Gone Haywire.* New York: Basic Books, 1997.

Gaynor, Mitchell L., and Jerry Hickey. *Dr. Gaynor's Cancer Prevention Program.* New York: Kensington, 1999.

Goldstein, Steven R., and Laurie Ashner. *The Estrogen Alternative.* New York: Putnam, 1998.

Hatherill, J. Robert. *Eat to Beat Cancer.* New York: St. Martin's Press, 1998.

Jacobowitz, Ruth S. *The Estrogen Answer Book.* Boston: Little, Brown, 1999.

Kent, Howard. *Breathe Better, Feel Better.* Peoples Medical Society, 1997.

Keon, Joseph. *The Truth About Breast Cancer: A 7-Step Prevention Program.* Mill Valley, CA: Parissound, 1999.

Keuneke, Robin. *Total Breast Health*. New York: Kensington, 1999.

Krohn, Jacqueline. *The Whole Way to Natural Detoxification*. Point Roberts, WA: Hartley & Marks, 1996.

Kushi, Michio. *The Macrobiotic Way. The Complete Macrobiotic Diet and Exercise Book*. Wayne, NJ: Avery, 1985.

Lee, John R. *Natural Progesterone: The Multiple Roles of a Remarkable Hormone*. Sebastopol, CA: BLL Publishing, 1993.

Lee, John R. *What Your Doctor May Not Tell You About Menopause*. New York: Warner Books, 1996.

Levenstein, Mary Kerney. *Everyday Cancer Risks and How to Avoid Them*. Garden City Park, NY: Avery Publishing, 1992.

Love, Susan M. *Dr. Susan Love's Breast Book*, 2nd ed. Reading, MA: Addison-Wesley Publishing, 1995.

Love, Susan M. *Dr. Susan Love's Hormone Book: Making Informed Choices About Menopause*. New York: Random House, 1997.

Lusk, Julie, ed. *30 Scripts for Relaxation, Imagery and Inner Healing*, 2 vols. Duluth, MN: Whole Person Associates, 1992.

Martin, Raquel. *The Estrogen Alternative*. Rochester, VT: Healing Arts Press, 1998.

McGinn, Kerry Anne. *The Informed Woman's Guide to Breast Health*. Palo Alto, CA: Bull Publishing, 1992.

Murray, Michael. *Encyclopedia of Natural Medicine*. Rocklin, CA: Prima Publishing, 1998.

Naparstek, Belleruth. *Staying Well with Guided Imagery: How to Harness the Power of Your Imagination for Health and Healing*. New York: Time/Warner, 1994.

Neifert, Marianne. *Dr. Mom's Guide to Breastfeeding*. New York: Penguin, 1998.

Northrup, Christiane. *Women's Bodies, Women's Wisdom*. New York: Bantam Books, 1994.

O'Donnell, Rosie, Tracy Chutorian Semler, and Deborah Axelrod. *Bosom Buddies: Lessons and Laughter on Breast Health and Cancer*. New York: Warner, 1999.

Robbins, John. *May All Be Fed*. New York: Avon, 1993.

Rogers, Sherry A. *Wellness Against All Odds*. Syracuse, NY: Prestige Publishing, 1994.

Rossman, Martin L. *Healing Yourself: A Step-by-Step Program for Better Health Through Imagery*. New York: Walker & Co., 1987.

Samuels, M., and N. Samuels. *Seeing with the Mind's Eye*. New York: Random House, 1981.

Siegel, Bernie S. *Peace, Love and Healing: Body-Mind Communication and the Path to Self-Healing*. New York: Harper & Row, 1989.

Singer, Sydney Ross, and Soma Grismaijer. *Dressed to Kill.* Garden City Park, NY: Avery Publishing, 1995.

Stone, Joanne, Keith Eddleman, and Mary Murray. *Pregnancy for Dummies.* Foster City, CA: IDG Books, 1999.

Stoppard, Miriam. *The Breast Book.* London: DK Publishing, 1996.

Tyler, Varro. *Herbs of Choice: The Therapeutic Use of Phytochemicals.* New York: Pharmaceutical Products Press, 1994.

Wade, Carlson. *Inner Cleansing.* West Nyack, NY: Parker Publishing, 1992.

Weed, Susun, and Christine Northrup. *Breast Cancer? Breast Health! The Wise Woman Way.* Ash Tree Publishing, 1997.

Weil, Andrew. *Natural Health, Natural Medicine: Eight Weeks to Optimum Health.* New York: Dorling Kindersley, 1994.

Werbach, Melvyn. *Healing Through Nutrition.* New York: Harper Collins, 1993.

Whitaker, Julian. *Dr. Whitaker's Guide to Natural Healing.* Rocklin, CA: Prima Publishing, 1995.

Wolfe, Honora Lee, and Bob Flaws. *Better Breast Health Naturally.* Blue Poppy, 1998.

Organizations

Breast-Feeding

International Childbirth Educators Association
P.O. Box 20048
Minneapolis, MN 55420
1-800-624-4934

La Leche League International
P.O. Box 1209
Franklin Park, IL 60131
1-800-525-3243

Breast Health Information

Breast Implant Information Network
1-800-887-6828
Hotline for information, newsletters

Cancer Information Service of the National Cancer Institute
1-800-4-CANCER

Cancer Research Council
4853 Cordell Avenue, Ste. 11
Bethesda, MD 20814
1-301-654-7933

Cancer Research Institute
681 Fifth Avenue
New York, NY 10022
1-800-99-CANCER
www.cancerresearch.org

Coping, Living with Cancer Magazine
P.O. Box 682268
Franklin, TN 37068-2268
e-mail:Copingmag@aol.com

ECAP (Exceptional Cancer Patients)
Bernie S. Siegel, M.D.
300 Plaza Middlesex
Middletown, CT 06457
1-860-343-5950

Meditation and Cancer
  Discussion Group
Hosted by HEALL at
www.heall.com

Michigan Breast Reconstruction
  Outcome Study
www.surg.med.umich.edu/plastic/
  breastrecon/brhtml

National Breast Cancer Coalition
1707 L Street NW, Ste. 160
Washington, DC 20036
1-202-296-7477
www.nbcc.org.au

National Cancer Institute
Building 31, Room 10 A 24
Bethesda, MD 20892
1-301-496-5583
1-800-422-6237 (cancer
  information specialist)

National Women's Health
  Network
13225 G St. NW
Washington, DC 20005

Simonton Cancer Center
P.O. Box 890
Pacific Palisades, CA 90272
1-310-459-4434

Susan G. Komen Breast Cancer
  Foundation
3005 LBJ Freeway, Suite 370
Dallas, TX 75244
1-214-980-8841
  or 1-800-IMAWARE
www.komen.org

Y-Me National Breast Cancer
  Organization
www.yme.org

Nutrition

American Dietetic Association
1-800-366-165
Recorded messages and live
  dietitians

American Institute for Cancer
  Research
1759 R Street NW
Washington, DC 10009
1-800-843-8114
www.aicr.org

Physicians Committee for
  Responsible Medicine
P.O. Box 6322
Washington, DC 20015
1-202-686-2210

Soy Protein Council
1255 23rd Street NW, Suite 850
Washington, DC 20037
1-202-467-6610
www.spcouncil.org

United Soybean Hotline
1-800-TALK SOY

Vegetarian Education Network
P.O. Box 3347
West Chester, PA 19380
1-215-696-VNET

Pesticides and Environmental Toxins

Center for Science in the Public
  Interest
1875 Connecticut Avenue NW,
  Ste. 300
Washington, DC 20009
1-202-332-9110

EMR Alliance
410 West 53rd Street, Ste. 402
New York, NY 10019
1-212-554-4073
e-mail: emrall@aol.com
Coalition concerned with electromagnetic fields

National Coalition Against the
  Misuse of Pesticides
701 E Street SE, Ste. 200
Washington, DC 20003
1-202-543-5450
www.ncamp.org

Rachel Carson Council
8940 Jones Mill Road
Chevy Chase, MD 20815
1-301-652-1877

Women's Environmental and
  Development Organization
845 Third Avenue
New York, NY 10022
1-212-759-7892

Risk Counseling

Strang Cancer Prevention Center
www.strang.org

Memorial Sloan-Kettering Cancer
  Center
www.mskcc.org

Specialists

The following organizations provide referrals for specialists:

American Association of Naturopathic Physicians
1-206-827-6035

American Cancer Society
1-800-ACS-2345

American College of Surgeons
1-312-202-5000

American Medical Association
1-312-464-5000

American Society of Plastic and
  Reconstructive Surgeons
1-800-635-0635

Therapies

Academy for Guided Imagery
P.O. Box 2070
Mill Valley, CA 94942
1-415-389-9324

American Massage Therapy Association
1-312-761-2682
For information on manual lymph
  drainage

International Association of Yoga
  Therapists
109 Hillside Avenue
Mill Valley, CA 94941
1-415-383-4587

North American Vodder Association of Lymphatic Therapy
P.O. Box 861
Chesterfield, OH 44026
1-216-729-3258

Stress Reduction Clinic
Jon Kabat-Zinn, Ph.D.
University of Massachusetts Medical Center
55 Lake Avenue North
Worcester, MA 01655
1-508-836-1616

Products for Breast Health

Diet

Natural coffee alternatives (for
  example, Yerba Mate, Postum,
  Pero Coffee, and others)
www.abundantearth.com
www.naturalpantry.com

Natural sweeteners: stevia
www.healthfree.com
www.mdvventures.com
www.stevia-rebaudiana-book.com

Exercise Videos

Better Than Before Fitness
Rehabilitation exercise video for
  breast cancer survivors
1-800-488-8354
jsforrest@breastfit.com
www.breastfit.com

Dare to Care
Videos for women recovering from
  breast cancer surgery
www.cancerfitness.com

Guided Imagery Tapes/Videos

Health Journeys, tapes by Belleruth
  Naparstek
2635 Payne Avenue
Cleveland, OH 44114
1-800-800-8661

Petrea King Collection
P.O. Box 190
Bundanoon, NSW 2578 Australia
www.PetreaKing.penrith.net.au

Source Cassette Learning Systems
P.O. Box W
Stanford, CA 94309
1-800-528-2737

MammaCare breast model and
  video
www.mammacare.com/
  mammacare.htm

Index